THE ULTIMATE GUIDE TO GETTING INTO PHYSICIAN ASSISTANT SCHOOL

Notice

Medicine is an ever-changing science. As new research and clinical experience broaden our knowledge, changes in treatment and drug therapy are required. The author and the publisher of this work have checked with sources believed to be reliable in their efforts to provide information that is complete and generally in accord with the standards accepted at the time of publication. However, in view of the possibility of human error or changes in medical sciences, neither the author nor the publisher nor any other party who has been involved in the preparation or publication of this work warrants that the information contained herein is in every respect accurate or complete, and they disclaim all responsibility for any errors or omissions or for the results obtained from use of the information contained in this work. Readers are encouraged to confirm the information contained herein with other sources. For example and in particular, readers are advised to check the product information sheet included in the package of each drug they plan to administer to be certain that the information contained in this work is accurate and that changes have not been made in the recommended dose or in the contraindications for administration. This recommendation is of particular importance in connection with new or infrequently used drugs.

THE ULTIMATE GUIDE TO GETTING INTO PHYSICIAN ASSISTANT SCHOOL

THIRD EDITION

Andrew J. Rodican, PA-C
Associate Medical Director
Medical Weight Loss Centers, LLC
East Haven, Connecticut

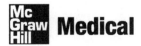

New York Chicago San Francisco Lisbon London Madrid Mexico City
Milan New Delhi San Juan Seoul Singapore Sydney Toronto

The Ultimate Guide to Getting into Physician Assistant School, Third Edition

4 5 6 7 8 9 0   DOC/DOC   14 13 12

ISBN 978-0-07-163973-6
MHID 0-07-163973-X

This book was set in Plantin by Aptara, Inc.
The editors were Joseph Morita and Regina Y. Brown.
The production supervisor was Catherine Saggese.
Production management was provided by Satvinder Kaur, Aptara, Inc.
The designer was Eve Siegel.
RR Donnelley was printer and binder.

This book is printed on acid-free paper.

Library of Congress Cataloging-in-Publication Data

Rodican, Andrew J.
    The ultimate guide to getting into physician assistant school / Andrew J. Rodican.—3rd ed.
       p. ; cm.
    Rev. ed. of: Getting into the physician assistant school of your choice. 2nd ed. c2004.
    Includes index.
    Summary: "The good news is that the Physician Assistant profession continues to thrive and grow. In fact, so many people are interested in the profession, competition to get into PA school may be even stiffer than medical school. Still, it is easy to see why many are choosing the PA profession. Medical students are flooded with $200,000 to $300,000 worth of debt after graduation and Medicare and insurance reimbursement rates are projected to decrease and threaten physician's income. In contrast, PA salaries continue to rise and opportunities are more prevalent than ever before. PAs continue to be "cost effective" for their employers"—Provided by publisher.
    ISBN-13: 978-0-07-163973-6 (pbk. : alk. paper)
    ISBN-10: 0-07-142185-8 (pbk. : alk. paper)
    1. Physicians' assistants—Education—United States.   2. Physicians' assistants—Vocational guidance.   3. Medical colleges—United States—Admission.   I. Rodican, Andrew J. Getting into the physician assistant school of your choice.   II. Title.
    [DNLM: 1. Physician Assistants—education—United States.   2. School Admission Criteria—United States.   3. Vocational Guidance—United States.   W 21.5 R692u 2011]
    R697.P45R646 2011
    610.73'72069071173—dc22

                                           2010016682

McGraw-Hill books are available at special quantity discounts to use as premiums and sales promotions, or for use in corporate training programs. To contact a representative please e-mail us at bulksales@mcgraw-hill.com.

This book is dedicated to the memory of my father,
James A. Rodican

About the Author

Andrew J. Rodican, PA-C, is a 1994 graduate of the Yale University School of Medicine Physician Associate Program. Rodican served on the admissions committee at Yale as both a student and an alumni member. He was also a recipient of the Yale University School of Medicine Physician Associate Program 1994 Medical Writing Award.

In 1996, Rodican self-published *The Ultimate Guide to Getting into Physician Assistant School* and formed the company AJR Associates, which is dedicated to helping PA school applicants navigate the admissions process through seminars and his coaching services.

Over the years, Rodican has worked in the fields of cardiothoracic surgery, occupational medicine, cardiology, and bariatric medicine. He is now the owner of Medical Weight Loss Centers in East Haven, Connecticut (www.MedWeightLossCenters.com).

Rodican's new PA school applicant Web site is www.andrewrodican.com, where applicants can find information and coaching or sign up for one of Rodican's seminars on getting into PA school.

Contents

Preface

At the time of this writing, the United States is facing multiple issues that concern the lives of all Americans. We are in a recession with no clear end in sight, our troops are involved in two wars with no end in sight, we are about to undergo major health care reform, and unemployment rates are greater than 10%. That's the bad news.

The good news is that the physician assistant profession continues to thrive and grow. In fact, so many people are interested in the profession, that competition to get into PA school may be even stiffer than that for medical school. Still, it is easy to see why many are choosing the PA profession. Medical students are flooded with $200,000 to $300,000 worth of debt after graduation, and Medicare and insurance reimbursement rates are projected to decrease and threaten physicians' income. In contrast, salaries for PAs continue to rise, and opportunities are more prevalent than ever. Moreover, PAs continue to be cost effective for their employers.

When I started my career as a cardiothoracic PA in 1994, I earned a salary of $46,000. In 2007, the average PA graduating from school earned a mean salary of $76,232, and the highest 90th percentile earned more than $90,000.

Today, I own my own practice, Medical Weight Loss Centers, and I have 20 employees who work for me. The beauty of the PA profession is that we have flexibility in where we practice, we've developed a solid reputation as quality health care providers, and we can practice medicine without carrying the heavy burden of debt acquired by so many medical students.

So, if you're thinking about becoming a PA or have definitive plans to apply to PA school, congratulations! You're making a wise decision that will pay dividends in ways you never imagined. Buckle up and enjoy the ride!

Andrew J. Rodican, PA-C

[CHAPTER 1]

So You Want to be a Physician Assistant

You will be asked many different times: "Why?" "Why do you want to become a physician assistant?" "Why don't you just go to medical school? You will make more money as a physician."

Your response to those questions and your final decision to apply to a physician assistant (PA) program will depend on how well you research answers to those same questions. This book can provide you with the information you need to answer such important questions.

No doubt, being a PA will challenge your intelligence, patience, compassion, and prejudices. But the profession will also reward you, not only financially but also emotionally. As you learn about the expanding roles for PAs in the medical field, you will realize how wonderfully versatile PAs are because of their "generalist" model of training. Upon graduation, you might start your first job in emergency medicine but later decide that you like surgery better. You can change specialties with an ease that physicians cannot. And you also will not have to manage the challenges that are associated with running a medical practice.

Your training will cost less than half that of a physician, and you can complete it in a little more than two years. Compare that to a physician's 4-year education and 3 or more years of postgraduation residency and fellowship. Can you put your life on hold for 8 to 12 years, or does 2 or 2.5 years sound better?

Competition for PA school positions is now more intense than the competition to get into medical school. Most PA programs require potential students to have a year or more of direct patient contact as a prerequisite. Often, applicants have worked as emergency room volunteers, patient care technicians, or medics on ambulances. Although a good grade point average is important, life experiences, maturity, and determination also make a good impression on admissions committees. Your personal essay should reflect all the influences that have brought you to the application process. Gather as much information as you can about the profession. And then this book will help you in your quest to prepare the best application possible.

FROM PETER THE GREAT TO POSTGRAD DEGREES

The Evolution of the PA Profession

The physician assistant profession has an amazingly long history. References to various military medical assistants go back as far as 1650 in the Russian army, led by Peter the Great. In the World War II era, Dr. Eugene Stead Jr. developed a curriculum model to fast-track the training of physicians in a 3-year time frame.

During the years from 1961 to 1972, the PA concept came more into focus when Dr. Stead established the first PA program at Duke University, in 1967. He used much the same model that he had used to train World War II physicians. He saw the need for midlevel health practitioners to complement the services and skills of physicians. This need was even more apparent in remote areas of the United States, where the medical profession had historically underserved populations. The opening of more PA programs during the ensuing period prompted the development of the PA professional organization, the American Academy of Physician Assistants (AAPA), in 1968. In 1970, Kaiser Permanente was the first health maintenance organization (HMO) to employ PAs. And in 1971, Montifiore Medical Center established the first PA postgrad surgical residency program.

In an effort to maintain consistency throughout PA programs, the American Medical Association's Committee on Allied Health Education and Accreditation developed training program guidelines in 1971 and implemented the program accreditation process. In 1973, the AAPA held its first conference. The first certifying exam was given in 1973, even before the National Commission on Certification of Physician Assistants (NCCPA) had been incorporated, in 1975.

The NCCPA was established to ensure the public that certified physician assistants meet established criteria and continue to meet those criteria every six years by taking a recertifying examination. The first recertification exam was given in 1981. Also, much state legislation has been implemented concerning the practice of PAs and their prescriptive privileges. National legislation also has been implemented to address PA reimbursement. By 1985, the ranks of PA had grown to more than 10,000 nationally, prompting the development of National PA Day in 1987. By 1988, the *Journal of the American Academy of Physician Assistants* was first published, complementing the field's first official journal publication in 1977, *Health Practitioner* (later called *Physician Assistant*).

In the 10 years after 1990, misconception and prejudices about PA privileges continued to fall away, allowing for an expanded role for PAs. The number of PA programs doubled. Discussion and implementation of master's-level programs began to take place. In 1993, there were 26,400 PAs in existence, but that number grew to 45,000 by 2002.

Presently, there are 149 PA programs in the United States. At the beginning of 2009, there were 79,706 PA graduates eligible to practice. There are many postgraduate residency programs in specialties as diverse as surgery, oncology, emergency medicine, psychology, otolaryngology, neonatology, and urology. The adoption of the PA model in many countries has also resulted in many new PAs. Those internationally trained PAs now represent their home countries at the annual AAPA conferences.

What is a Physician Assistant?

Physician assistants are health care professionals licensed to practice medicine with physician supervision. Rather than follow their physician colleagues around by their proverbial coattails, most PAs work autonomously and collaboratively with their physician supervisors. Moreover, PAs are trained as generalists and perform various duties depending on the specialty, practice setting, supervising physician, and scope of practice. In general, PAs are trained to perform a comprehensive history and physical examination, to formulate a diagnosis and treatment plan, to order and interpret diagnostic tests, to assist in surgery, to prescribe medications, to counsel patients and their families, to perform minor surgical procedures, and to consult with their supervising physicians.

There are PAs in more than 60 different areas and specialties of medical and surgical practice. About half of all PAs work in primary care (e.g., family practice, obstetrics and gynecology, pediatric and internal medicine). Another 20% work in various surgical subspecialties, and the remainder of PAs work in a host of other specialty and subspecialty areas, administration, and research. Some PAs actually own their own practice and hire a supervising physician to work for them.

The average PA is 41 years old, and the profession is almost equally divided among men and women. A new graduate can earn approximately $76,232 per year in the first year. The average PA earns between $85,710 and $89,987 per year. Many PAs, depending on experience and scope of practice, earn more than $100,000 per year.

Another interesting trend in the PA profession is the move away from 2-year undergraduate certificate programs to full master's-level programs. In 2007, 40% of students graduated with a BA/BS-level PA degree. Another 43% held master's-level PA diplomas. There is also a trend toward the awarding of doctorates of PA studies. Currently, about 4% of PAs work as PA educators. Many of those people have already acquired a Ph.D. in a related health care discipline, which gives them credibility as professional educators in the many PA programs that have emerged in the past 20 years.

How are PAs Trained?

The length of PA programs varies from 24 months to 32 months, depending on whether it is an undergraduate or a master's-level program. Of the programs, 80% award a master's degree, 113 award master's degrees, 21 award bachelor's degrees, 3 award associate degrees, and 5 award certificates.

Students are trained in the medical model, similar to that of most medical school programs. In fact, the didactic phase (first year) of a PA program is often equated to the first three years of medical school. Many PAs share some classes with medical students in programs that are affiliated with a medical school. The main difference between physician training and PA training is the number of years a physician is required to spend in a residency after the didactic phase is completed.

The first year of a PA program is typically five full days and sometimes 1 or 2 evenings per week of classroom and clinical practicum sessions. Students can expect to take first-year courses in clinical laboratory services, electrocardiography, emergency medicine and trauma, interviewing techniques, medicine, general surgery, microbiology and infectious diseases, pharmacology, physical examination, anatomy and physiology, biochemistry, psychodynamics of human behavior, diagnostic imaging, epidemiology and public health, human sexuality, medical ethics, and pathology.

The second year is geared toward clinical rotations. Most programs have mandatory rotations in emergency medicine, family or general medicine, general surgery, microbiology and infectious diseases, pharmacology, physical examinations, internal medicine, obstetrics and gynecology, pediatrics, geriatric medicine, orthopedics, and psychiatry. In addition, students can typically choose from a number of elective rotations. In programs that offer master's degrees, students are required to complete clinical research and a thesis paper.

On graduating from an accredited PA program, students are eligible to sit for the national certifying exam, the Physician Assistant National Certifying Exam, which is a multiple-choice test that comprises 360 questions that assess basic medical and surgical knowledge. The NCCPA administers the test in conjunction with the National Board of Medical Examiners. Students are eligible for state licensure after they pass this national examination. To maintain certification, PAs must document 100 hours of continuing medical education (CME) every two years and pass a national recertifying exam every 6 years.

What is the Future of the PA Profession?

To project the future of the PA profession, we must first look at the changes in the past 10 years in the health care industry. More than $1.2 trillion is spent annually on health care. Everyone is aware of the drive for efficiency in health care delivery and the push to cut costs at the same time. More than 80% of Americans are enrolled in managed care plans, including HMOs and preferred provider organizations (PPOs). More than 53% of practicing PAs are primary care providers, who also provide patient education, prevention, and wellness as part of their job.

The PA profession has benefited from two major changes in health care delivery. First, in 2003, the Accreditation Council for Graduate Medical Education, the American Osteopathic Association, and most states established limitations on house-staff duty hours (the hours that interns and residents can work). This effectively reduced by up to 25% the amount of inpatient coverage provided by house staff per patient. Because most house doctors (those who are available in the hospital to admit and follow patients) were typically interns and residents, this new policy reducing their hours affected hospitals greatly. Many hospital administrators saw that PAs could replace residents and interns, and PAs became the right people in the right place at the right time (at the right price) to fill these positions.

Second, community-based attending physicians were not being adequately reimbursed for hospital rounds, so they began allowing their patients to be followed by the hospitalists, the in-house physician, resident, or physician assistant. This allowed attending physicians to stay in their office, which was more cost-effective because they could see more patients and get better reimbursed. Thus, there was an increase in the need for hospitalists—a role that many PAs had begun to fill.

It is easy, then, to see why the Bureau of Labor Statistics has rated the PA profession as twelfth fastest-growing occupation in the period from 2000 to 2010.

How can I Stand Out as a PA School Applicant?

Because the application process is very competitive, applicants should satisfy all prerequisites before applying. One of the most common questions the admissions board asks is, If we have only one position left to fill, why should we pick you? Also, while grades and test scores are important, but so is clinical experience, maturity, and life experience. The board will question your level of commitment. If you see PA school as a stepping-stone to medical school, you will quickly be weeded out because they are interested in applicants who want to be a PA, not a physician. The committee also wants applicants who understand the concept and believe in the mission of being a PA.

As you read through this book, you will begin to understand five qualities that will make you a very strong candidate. As you build on these qualities, you will become a confident and qualified PA school applicant.

CHAPTER 2

What Do PA Programs Look for in Applicants?

Luck is when preparedness meets opportunity.

—Author unknown

At the time of this writing, there are 149 accredited PA programs in the United States. If you were to interview admissions committee members from each program, you would probably get 149 different opinions and ideas on what committees look for in PA school applicants. Fortunately, there are some basic criteria that all programs follow to evaluate candidates for admission. The five basic categories include the following:

1. Passion
2. Academic ability and test scores
3. Medical experience
4. Understanding of the PA profession
5. Maturity

In this chapter, we consider each of those five categories.

PASSION

Passion is the fuel that can propel an otherwise-average candidate to the top of the applicant pool. Passion is the burning desire that motivates an applicant to study that extra hour, take that additional chemistry course, or gain that extra year of hands-on medical experience before applying to PA school. **Passion takes the words *I can't* and replaces them with *I will*.** Passion cannot be taught; it must come from deep within.

If you have a passion for being a PA, you will take certain steps on your own. You will find the time to locate and shadow PAs in your community. You will read PA journals and become aware of issues and trends in the PA profession. You will understand what the PA role is all about and will be able to verbalize exactly why you want to become a PA rather than a physician or a nurse-practitioner.

A key benefit of having passion is the motivation it provides. On Saturday nights, when you would prefer to be out with your friends rather than studying pharmacology or microbiology, your passion will keep you focused. On clinical rotations, when you are spending nights in the on-call room rather than sleeping in your own bed, your passion for practical experience will make it all seem worthwhile.

The admissions committee can sense your passion from your essay or from simply looking you in the eye at the interview. Think about why you really want to become a PA, and try to incorporate that passion into the entire application process.

ACADEMIC ABILITY AND TEST SCORES

Applicants to PA school frequently want to know the magic grade point average (GPA) or entrance exam score needed to gain acceptance to a PA program. Many applicants falsely assume that they must possess a 4.0 GPA and 1,500 SAT scores to be competitive candidates. That simply isn't true. In fact, the average applicant probably falls somewhere between a 3.0 and 3.2 GPA, with SAT scores in the 1,000 to 1,100 range.

It is important, though, that a candidate demonstrates a reasonable aptitude in the hard sciences. Ultimately, the committee will want to be sure that you can manage an academically challenging program that encompasses graduate-level coursework in anatomy and physiology, biochemistry, and the pathophysiology of the disease process. If you had a difficult time with undergraduate chemistry and biology, you will surely struggle in PA school. Competition is intense, and although the committee may overlook a grade of C in U.S. history or Spanish, it will be less tolerant of a marginal grade in the sciences.

Table 2.1. High School Science Scores

Year in School	Mary	Bob
Freshman	General Chemistry: D+ Microbiology: C	General Chemistry: A Microbiology: A
Sophomore	Organic Chemistry: C Biochemistry: B	Organic Chemistry: A Biochemistry: B
Junior	Inorganic Chemistry: B Cell Biology: A	Inorganic Chemistry: B Cell Biology: C
Senior	Physical Chemistry: A Genetics: A	Physical Chemistry: D+ Genetics: C

The good news is that committees consider trends rather than absolute numbers. For instance, undergraduate students who have a few Cs, or even a D, as freshmen can make a favorable impression on a committee if they rebounded with As and Bs in their junior and senior years. In fact, students who continue to improve will fare much better than students who trend downward.

To further illustrate the point, let's look at Table 2.1, which shows the undergraduate science grades of two hypothetical applicants, Mary and Bob.

Both applicants have an identical GPA, approximately 3.0, yet Mary's overall trend is upward, whereas Bob's trend is downward. Mary would be the stronger candidate with respect to academic performance.

Other factors the committee considers when evaluating a candidate's academic ability include the number of credit hours per semester, course difficulty, reputation of the college or university, life's difficulties and circumstances, and extracurricular activities. Let's look at each of these factors separately.

Number of Credit Hours per Semester

A typical day in PA school may require students to sit in the classroom for 8 to 10 hours, attend an early evening physical examination seminar, and study for 3 to 4 more hours that night in preparation for a pharmacology exam the following morning. This rigorous daily schedule demands excellent time-management skills from students, as well as an ability to comprehend and assimilate volumes of scientific material. The only means the admissions committee has to evaluate whether you can make the grade in this area is by reviewing your undergraduate transcript. Applicants who carried a full undergraduate course load while working part-time will make more favorable impressions on the committee than applicants who took fewer classes or didn't work at all.

Course Difficulty

The admissions committee will probably favor the application from a chemistry major who achieved a 3.0 GPA over that of a history major who achieved a higher GPA of 3.3. This fact should not be surprising to most applicants. It is the committee's job to select those applicants who are best suited to thrive in a graduate-level science program.

Reputation of the College or University

Although the area of a college or university's reputation is highly subjective, the learning institution itself can be a deciding factor in the application process. For example, let's consider two applicants in the running for the last available slot in a class. Mark has a 3.0 GPA in biochemistry from Harvard University. John has an overall 3.7 GPA in biology from a state university, but he also took many of his undergraduate prerequisite science courses at the local community college before transferring to the state university. John's GPA is higher, but Mark will probably be accepted because of the strength and reputation of his undergraduate institution.

Life's Difficulties and Circumstances

We all experience a variety of trauma in our lives, and some of us more than others. The committee will certainly consider unusual circumstances that may have influenced your GPA or other areas of your application. Significant stressors may include divorce, death of a significant other, or a serious medical illness. Although you cannot avoid special circumstances and the committee will consider each case individually, it is important to demonstrate how you may have overcome your particular challenge or obstacle and to indicate that you are now focused on your goal.

Extracurricular Activities

Grades aren't everything. Admissions committees look for well-rounded individuals with quality life experience. Be sure to let the committee know if you volunteered in the Peace Corps, if you play in a band, or even if you race motorcycles. Life experience is an invaluable resource to you as a medical professional. Physician assistants must be able to relate to patients from varied cultures and backgrounds.

Standardized Test Scores

Suffice it to say that SAT and GRE scores are prerequisites for most programs, but they do not play a significant role in the admissions process. Standardized test scores come into play only if you've scored exceptionally high or extremely low, and they serve to validate the rest of your application.

MEDICAL EXPERIENCE

Applicants to PA school, and especially strong applicants, come to the table with a variety of medical experience. Unfortunately, some applicants have no medical experience at all, which certainly hurts their chances of acceptance. Most committee members will insist on some prior medical experience before they will consider an applicant as a serious candidate.

On average, four years of prior experience in one of the following areas is common:

- **Nursing**
  - Registered nurse (RN)
  - Licensed practical nurse (LPN)
  - Certified nursing assistant (CNA)
- **Allied Health**
  - Physical therapist
  - Occupational therapist
  - X-ray technician
- **Emergency Services**
  - Emergency medical technician (EMT)
  - Paramedic
  - Emergency room technician
- **Miscellaneous**
  - Phlebotomist

- ○ Athletic trainer
- ○ Medical researcher
- ○ Medical volunteer

As mentioned repeatedly in this text, applying to PA school is an extremely competitive process. The more points you score with a committee, the better your chances are. Think about your own experience and how you might be able to improve on it. If you have little or no medical experience, consider doing volunteer work at the local hospital or clinic. **The more hands-on medical experience you have, the stronger you will be as a candidate.**

UNDERSTANDING OF THE PA PROFESSION

The PA profession has enjoyed tremendous growth over the past decade. That trend, according to the U.S. Bureau of Labor Statistics, is expected to continue for at least another decade. In fact, CNNMoney.com has noted that demand for PAs will increase by more than 27% in the coming ten years and ranked the profession among the top ten for job growth. *Money* magazine ranked PAs second in its list of the best jobs, which looked at well-paying and good jobs. Salaries for PAs are at an all-time high and continue to rise. According to the American Academy for Physician Assistants, the median PA salary in 2008 was $89,987. As a result of these positive factors, applications to the various PA programs remain strong. The challenge facing admissions committees is to separate the wheat from the chaff, if you will. One way committee members do this is by closely examining all applicants' motivation for becoming a PA and deciding whether they have a realistic understanding of the PA profession.

Many applicants view PA school as a stepping-stone to medical school. This is a huge mistake. Although both professions allow the individual to practice medicine, PAs do not want to be MDs; they want to be PAs. The MD wannabe who becomes a PA first will be miserable, and the committee will see right through that tactic.

Before you apply to become a PA, be sure you understand what it means to be a dependent practitioner. In other words, unlike nurse-practitioners, PAs must always work under the direct supervision of a physician. This does not mean that you will follow your supervising physician around by the coattails, however. In fact, PAs are expected to be fairly autonomous with respect to evaluating and treating their own patients. What this does mean, though, is that you will have a physician available to assist you with more difficult and complex cases. This is actually a nice benefit of being a PA.

To get a better understanding of the PA profession, try shadowing various PAs who work in different specialties. Most PAs will be excited about your interest in the profession and will gladly have you follow them as they perform their duties.

MATURITY

The mean age of a PA is 41. However, the maturity the screening committee looks for in an applicant doesn't necessarily have anything to do with age. The committee member who reviews your application is well aware that you will likely have a patient's life in your hands on any given day. **You must demonstrate maturity through your prior work experience, in your essay, and at the interview.** Some basic questions the committee will want answered to determine your maturity include the following:

- Can you be empathetic, yet assertive?
- Can you handle stress under fire?
- Will you know when to call for help?
- Do you exhibit good judgment?
- Can you make quick decisions?
- Are you a self-starter?
- Will you require constant supervision?

PA school applicants come from diverse backgrounds and possess a variety of life experiences. Some of the most interesting candidates have careers that are totally unrelated to health care at the time of application. A typical applicant pool may include an attorney, a schoolteacher, and an actress among its ranks. Students may range in age from 21 to 61. The common trait that most mature applicants share is the ability to exhibit a youthful energy coupled with practical life experience.

Now that you have a better understanding of exactly what committees look for in an applicant, let's see if we can come up with a specific plan for you to achieve this worthy goal.

CHAPTER 3

Setting Goals

Whatever the mind of man can conceive and believe, it can achieve.

—Napoleon Hill (Author of Think and Grow Rich)

WHY SET GOALS?

Few people bother to set realistic goals in life. Most people are what Zig Ziglar, in his video *Goals: Setting and Achieving Them on Schedule,* calls "wandering generalit[ies]" but need to become "meaningful specific[s]." The bottomline is that the competition for admission to PA school is fierce. **Without a written goal, a plan of action, and the ability to focus, your chances of being accepted to the program of your choice are slim.**

The basic problem most people have with setting goals is not time, but a lack of direction. Everyone has the same 24 hours to work with each day. Why is it that some people achieve so much, while others who are equally intelligent and capable can't seem to accomplish anything? The former have goals—written, measurable, and realistic goals—and they know how to achieve them. Numerous authors, from Stephen Covey to Norman Vincent Peale, have discussed how to go about setting goals. Many people agree that specific long- and short-term goals will lead you to become more creative, which will, in turn, add more excitement and fulfillment to your life.

Do you know why 97% of people never really set goals in the proper fashion? As Zig Ziglar says, the answer is fear, or "false evidence appearing real." But what are we afraid of? Some of us are afraid of failure. Some of us fear the competition. Some of us are afraid of success. After all, there is danger in setting goals—we might actually achieve them! We've all heard the phrase "be careful what you wish for."

But there is more danger in not setting goals, especially the danger of wasting your resources. As they say, a boat in dry dock rots more quickly than a boat at sea. Don't waste your resources, and write down your goals today (see Appendix C).

If I haven't yet convinced you of the importance of goal setting, perhaps this next story will. In 1953, a study at Yale University polled graduating seniors about how many of them had written goals and a plan of action for carrying out those goals. Surprisingly, only 3% of Yale students had a complete plan—10% had taken some steps, and 87% had set no goals at all and had no plan of action for life after graduation. Those people are wandering generalities.

In 1973, twenty years later, the university polled those same seniors again. This time researchers asked them about their successes in measurable areas: finances, career, and position in life. Not surprisingly, the 3% of graduates who had set goals and had written a plan of action to carry them out had accomplished more than the other 97% of graduates combined.

SEVEN-STEP FORMULA FOR SUCCESS

If you learn the following seven-step formula for success, it won't make a difference what your goals are. You will be able to accomplish them. By knowing and following the seven steps, you will maximize your chances of getting into the PA school of your choice:

1. Identify the goal.
2. Set a deadline for achievement.
3. List obstacles to overcome.
4. Identify people and organizations that can help you.
5. List the skills and knowledge required to achieve your goal.
6. Develop a plan of action.
7. List the benefits of achieving the goal, and ask yourself, "What's in it for me?"

Now take out a pencil and paper and begin listing your goals. If you do nothing else with this book, you will at least have completed a goal sheet. If you need some help getting started, take a look at my written goal statement about PA school in 1992. You'll notice that I wrote out my goals in paragraph form, but write your goals however you prefer. The point is to get started with the writing.

August 15, 1990

By May 1, 1992 I will be accepted into Yale, University of Florida, or Wake Forest's Bowman Gray's Physician Assistant Program. To accomplish this goal, I first have to discuss my desire to become a PA with my wife and convince her that this is the right thing to do for our family. Next, I need to begin saving money so that I can help my wife support our two children and provide food and shelter for the next two years. Finally, I will stay focused and not listen to those people who will say I'm crazy or having an early midlife crisis for wanting to quit a great job at age 35 and go back to school for 2 years.

I will immediately contact the American Academy of Physician Assistants (AAPA) and the Connecticut Academy of Physician Assistants (ConnAPA) to find out what resources are available to me. I will get a PA programs directory and begin writing to several schools, focusing on my top three choices. I will contact the president of ConnAPA and get to know him. I will also visit Yale's PA program and visit with Elaine Grant, who is the dean of the program, and maintain contact with her quarterly. I will do the same thing at the other two programs. I will find out from those people what I lack as a competitive candidate and how I can best strengthen my application.

I will visit with some PAs who work in my wife's office and spend as much time with them as possible (shadowing). I will attend as many open houses as possible to learn more about each program and to make myself known to them.

I will need to take courses in anatomy and physiology (I and II) and microbiology to fulfill requirements (prerequisites). I will achieve no less than an A in each class. I will also begin volunteering at Saint Raphael's hospital, in the emergency room, to gain more "current" experience. I will also obtain an SAT study guide to prepare myself for the test, which I need to take to get into Yale.

My plan is to continue working full-time, save money, and do volunteer work part-time. I will also take evening classes. While working in a hospital, I will discuss my goals with as many PAs as possible and learn as much as I can about the PA profession.

Once I achieve my goal of getting into the PA school of my choice, I will enjoy many benefits: helping people, job satisfaction, secure future, challenging work, stimulating work, prestige, a sense of accomplishment, and much more.

I wrote those goals in 1990. I can also vividly remember the exact moment I decided to apply to PA school. I was on vacation with my family in Orlando, Florida. I was in the office of my friend Chuck Ruotolo looking through the classifieds when I spotted a job opening for a plastic surgery PA. On a whim, I called the number and spoke with the office secretary. She practically begged me to come in for an interview. In my excitement, I forgot to tell her that I wasn't a PA at all, but I didn't want to spoil her enthusiasm. It was at that exact moment that I told my friend Chuck I was going to become a PA. He said, "Go for it!" and I have never looked back.

Twelve years later, I am entering my 16th year as a PA. As I sit writing the third edition to this book, I now realize that the moment in Orlando was one of the turning points in my life. I have never regretted my decision to become a PA. I've enjoyed all of the benefits I listed on my goal sheet and many more than I could have imagined at that time.

Here's another example of an applicant who, having put a hurried application together for PA school and failed to get in, reassessed his priorities and concentrated on new goals:

I planned for things to be different next year. I would do the following:
- Identify schools I could apply to using the Association of PA Programs (APAP) directory of PA programs.
- Apply to at least five new schools to increase the opportunity of being interviewed.
- Request and complete a school's application as soon as it was available.
- Type and proofread everything I sent to the program.
- Join the AAPA as an affiliate member.
- Visit as many programs as I could during a summer trip east.
- Continue to take classes that would prepare me for PA school.

By the end of the year, I had applied to nine schools. I had attended one interview and had three more after the first year. To prepare for those, I read several interview books and bought a new suit. I studied up on some of the issues facing the profession and health care in general. I tried to relax. The interviews were similar in format, as were the questions. Then I had to wait. Two weeks after the last interview, I was notified by my top choice that I was accepted. The years of going to school during the day and working at night, the preparation for the interviews, and the trips across the country had all paid off. I was in.

IMAGING

Once you have determined your goals, it is important to imagine them being accomplished. Imaging is a technique that I learned in Officer Training School while becoming an officer in the U.S. Air Force. Imaging is a powerful tool. The epigraph to this chapter— "Whatever the mind of man can conceive and believe, it can achieve"—is a true statement.

To test out imaging, try to get a crystal-clear image of yourself performing well at the interview for PA school. You are calm and relaxed. Picture yourself going to the mailbox and opening that acceptance letter. Each day spend a little time thinking about your goal until it becomes an obsession for you. You'll be surprised at the results. When I was thinking about getting into a PA program, I would spend a half hour every day visualizing my goal while I was on my exercise machine. I had a perfect image of the acceptance letter, right down to the color of the school's logo. I would get myself worked up into a frenzy just thinking about it. I've calculated that I spent about 180 hours imaging.

Guess what? My efforts paid off. I interviewed at the University of Florida in December 1991, on a Friday. The next Monday I received a phone call from the program congratulating me on my acceptance. I also was accepted to Yale's program in March 1992. I chose to stay local and go to Yale. I also received an invitation to interview at Wake Forest's Bowman Gray in North Carolina. **I achieved my goal of getting into the PA school of my first choice (Yale) by having a written goal, working hard, and simply carrying out my written plan of action.**

TAKE A PERSONAL EVALUATION

In addition to setting goals and imaging with positive outcomes, it is also necessary to review your performance and evaluate those areas in which you need improvement. Going to PA school can be a major life transition, and before you jump in to the water, it's a good idea to take a personal inventory, if you will. The best way to start this inventory is to look at seven specific areas of your life, Every so often, evaluate yourself with respect to the following seven areas and ask yourself some questions:

1. Appearance: Do I present myself well? Do I need to lose some weight or buy a new pair of shoes for the interview?
2. Family: Is my family supportive of my goal? Will this career change cause conflict in my family life? Am I willing to listen to the skeptics, and will I follow my dream unconditionally?
3. Financial: Can I afford to go to PA school now? Does the school offer graduate-level student loans? Can I save enough money between now and the time school starts?
4. Social: Am I a team player? Am I willing to practice medicine as a dependent practitioner?
5. Spiritual: Is it morally right for me to do this now? Do I have other obligations or responsibilities? Am I being selfish?
6. Mental: Should I take any additional courses or retake any courses? Am I well read on medical issues and current events? Will I have many distractions?
7. Career: Do I really know why I want to become a PA versus a physician or a nurse-practitioner? Do I fully understand the role of the PA?

Score your answers in these seven areas on a scale from 1 to 5, with 5 being the highest and 1 being the lowest. Be honest with yourself. Work on those areas in which you score low. Taking this personal inventory will keep you focused and help you reach your goals more quickly.

SET BIG GOALS

There once were two men, one old and one young, fishing on a pier. The young man watched as the older man kept reeling in big fish but throwing them back into the water. "Why are you throwing back those big, beautiful fish?" asked the young man. "Because I only have this little frying pan," replied the old man, holding up a scrawny little skillet.

Without big goals, you will never accomplish great things. The old fisherman was a great fisherman, but his skillet—his goal—was too small. Dig down deep into your soul and focus on what you want in life. Make a plan and envision yourself accomplishing each task. Ralph Waldo Emerson once wrote, "What lies behind us and what lies before us are tiny matters compared to what lies within us."

WITH WHOM DO I SHARE MY GOALS?

We can think about goals in two ways. Some goals are "give-up" goals, goals that are designed around letting go or getting rid of something. For example, if you want to lose (or give up) twenty pounds, then let everybody at home and at the office know about it.

In contrast, a "go-up" goal is a goal designed to get you something—a new job, more financial security, and so on. Getting into PA school is a go-up goal. Share go-up goals only with your closest friends and family, as they're the ones who are most likely to support you. You can easily be derailed if you share your go-up goals with people who won't support the goal. Before you tell someone about your plan to go to PA school, ask yourself the following question: "Will this person support me in this goal?" If the answer is no, think twice about sharing your important goal with that person.

GETTING FOCUSED

I'd like to touch a bit on the power of focus. Just because you've decided to apply to PA school does not mean that life stops happening. You still will have to deal with the daily stressors that life throws your way, like finding enough time to research schools and fill out applications, taking additional courses (if necessary), balancing your business and family life, and managing financial pressures. Some applicants may find it too overwhelming to deal with all of those issues and decide to throw in the towel. Before you find yourself in that position, know that it is absolutely normal to feel overwhelmed at times. All of us have felt the same way. In fact, I often felt overwhelmed during PA school, but I learned some techniques that helped me to survive and thrive. I would like to pass on one of those techniques with you right now.

List Your Top 25 Goals

In this chapter, I asked you to consider setting goals in seven specific areas: appearance, family, financial, social, spiritual, mental, and career. Because this book is about getting into PA school, I focus on career goals, specifically as they relate to applying to PA school. Keep in mind, however, that this technique I am about to share with you works for all seven areas.

The first thing to do is list 25 goals, right off the top of your head, which you need to accomplish to be a strong applicant for PA school. To do this properly, you need the brochures and information on each of the schools you are applying to. Write down everything you will need to do, in no particular order. For example, if you plan to apply to PA school in one year, your list may look like this:

1. Prepare for entrance exams.
2. Take entrance exams.
3. Take microbiology course at local college.
4. Find three PAs to shadow.
5. Gain one more year of hands-on experience.
6. Start working on essay.
7. Locate three people who will write a letter of reference for me.
8. Join the AAPA as an affiliate member.
9. Join my state chapter of the AAPA as an affiliate member.
10. Save $50 per week to augment my income while in school.
11. Locate and speak with three graduated PAs from the schools I am applying to.
12. Attend each school's open house.
13. Schedule a phone conversation with each school's director.
14. Request applications from each school I am applying to.
15. Find out dates entrance exams are given.
16. Register for microbiology class.
17. Contact volunteer offices at local hospitals.
18. Fill out applications.
19. Send for college transcripts and send to each PA program.
20. Learn about the history of each program that I am applying to.
21. Buy a new suit for the interview.
22. Create a file for each program with application deadlines on the cover.
23. Attend a meeting of the state chapter of the AAPA.
24. Search the Internet for sites relevant to PA school applicants.
25. Be able to talk about five current issues facing the PA profession.

If you can list more than 25 goals, by all means, do so. I know that the list can be overwhelming at times. Relax, though, because I am going to show you how to prioritize your list and make it very manageable.

Prioritize the List

Now that you have listed everything you need to do before you become a strong PA school applicant, the next step is to prioritize. Take a look at each one of your 25 goals and determine a realistic time frame for you to accomplish them.

Beside each goal write a number—3, 6, 9, or 12 months. This will give you a general time frame to work from. For example, if you need to take the entrance exams before you apply to PA school, you will probably place a 3 next to goal No. 15, "Find out dates entrance exams are given," because you may want to take the entrance exams twice to ensure that the schools see your best score. You also want to be sure that you have plenty of time to take the entrance exams and get the scores to the appropriate PA programs before their application deadline. However, you will probably place a 12 next to goal No. 21, because buying a new suit for the interview is likely to be one of the last things you'll need to do.

The NCAA Tournament Draw

The next step is to list all of your 3s on the left-hand side of a clean sheet of paper. As an example, I chose eight 3s from the previous list as follows:

1. Prepare for entrance exams.
2. Take entrance exams.
3. Join AAPA.
4. Join state chapter of AAPA.
5. Save $50 per week.
6. Request applications from PA schools.
7. Find out entrance exam dates.
8. Register for microbiology class.

Now place these goals in a format similar to what newspapers publish during the NCAA basketball tournament in March of each year.

Format for NCAA-Type Bracket

Round 1	Round 2	Round 3	Winner
1. Take entrance exams	Find out entrance exam dates		
2. Find out entrance exam dates		Find out entrance exam dates	
3. Join AAPA	Join state chapter of AAPA		
4. Join state chapter of AAPA			
5. Save $50 per week			Register for microbiology course
	Request PA school applications		
6. Request PA school applications		Register for microbiology course	
7. Prepare for entrance exams	Register for microbiology course		
8. Register for microbiology course			

Instead of placing eight college basketball teams in the left-hand column, you substitute your 3-month goals for getting into PA school. Then you decide which goal moves on to the next round according to the significance you place on that goal in comparison with the others. In our example, registering for a microbiology class wins because there may be only two semesters in which you can take the course. If you do not complete the course before the PA school's application deadline, you probably won't have a chance of being accepted. Therefore, by the process of elimination, you would choose registering for a microbiology class as your primary goal to accomplish in the following three months.

Once you accomplish your primary goal (or priority), you can work backward until you have accomplished all of your 3-month goals. You can make up a similar format for your 6-, 9-, and 12-month goals. By following the format for each time frame, you will be able to stay focused on your top priorities. You will also eliminate the frustration and chaos that sometimes can be overwhelming when you don't know what to do next.

Wow! We've covered a lot in this chapter. The important takeaway message in this chapter is to set big goals, write them down, follow the seven-step formula for success, and use the NCAA tournament method to prioritize your list and help you focus. There—that wasn't too difficult. Now get started!

[CHAPTER 4]

Selecting a Program

It is your work in life that is the ultimate seduction.

—Pablo Picasso

All physician assistant programs are not created equally. Many programs have a primary care focus, and a few have a surgical focus. Many programs offer a master's degree, and others offer a graduate certificate, bachelor's degree, or an associate's degree. Most programs average two years in length, but some are longer. Tuition varies from a few thousand dollars at some programs to more than $20,000 at others. Some programs are affiliated with a medical school, but others are not. Some programs favor applicants from their home state. Why spend a great deal of energy and money applying to a particular school only to find out later that you aren't really a good fit for that particular program? In this chapter, I give you some food for thought to consider before you apply to any PA program.

Before we go into the details of programs, I encourage you to join the American Academy of Physician Assistants (AAPA) as an affiliate member, as well as your state chapter affiliate of the AAPA (see Appendix E). Joining these professional associations is critical to understanding different programs. To join the AAPA, call or write:

American Academy of Physician Assistants
950 N. Washington Street
Alexandria, VA 22314-1552
Phone: (703) 836-2272
Fax: (703) 684-1924
E-mail: aapa@aapa.org
Web: www.aapa.org

ACCREDITATION

When deciding which program(s) to apply to, your first order of business is to consider the accreditation status of the program. You will want to attend a program that is accredited by the Commission on Accreditation of Allied Health Education Programs. The Accreditation Review Committee on Education for the Physician Assistant includes representatives from the American Medical Association, the Association of Physician Assistant Programs (APAP), the American Academy of Family Physicians, the American Academy of Pediatrics, the American College of Physicians, and the American College of Surgeons. According to data obtained from the Physician Assistant Educator Association, there were 147 accredited PA programs in the United States as of fall 2009.

If you do not graduate from an accredited PA program, you will not be eligible to sit for the national certifying examination for physician assistants, which is administered by the National Commission on Certification of Physician Assistants (NCCPA). Without your NCCPA certification, you will not be eligible for state licensure and won't be able to practice in most locations.

If you are applying to a relatively new program, check to make sure that it has a provisional accreditation status, which means that it has received a comprehensive evaluation prior to opening. Although the provisional status does not guarantee later accreditation, at least you can get an idea of where the program stands in the accreditation process.

If you have any questions or concerns relative to accreditation issues, contact:

NCCPA
12000 Findley Road
Suite 200
Duluth, GA 30097

Phone: 678-417-8100
Fax: 678-417-8135
Email: nccpa@nccpa.net

FOCUS OF THE PROGRAM

Most admissions committees select applicants on the basis of several criteria that include but are not limited to academics, test scores (e.g., SAT,

GRE, AHPAT, TOEFL), understanding of the PA profession and concept, health care experience, volunteer work, community service, interviews, the narrative statement (essay), and personal or professional references. Certain programs, however, mention a particular focus for their selection criteria (e.g., primary care, in-state residents, surgical). It is important to know the focus of various programs so that you apply to those that are the best fit with your qualifications and goals.

The Association of Post Graduate PA Programs has identified programs that specifically mention a focus in the section on selection factors in their application or brochure. Keep in mind that these factors are not always absolute criteria, and applicants should always consult with individual programs for an idea of the significance of each one.

Practice in Underserved Areas

Augsburg College

City University of New York, Harlem Hospital Center

Drexel University

Lock Haven University

Oregon Health Sciences University

Riverside Community College

University of California, Davis

Stanford University

University of North Dakota School of Medicine

University of Oklahoma, Tulsa

University of Southern California School of Medicine

University of Texas

University of Utah School of Medicine

University of Washington

University of Wisconsin–Madison

Cardiothoracic Surgery

Methodist DeBakey Heart Center

St. Josephy Mercy Hospital Cardiothoracic Surgery Program
Critical Care

Johns Hopkins Hospital Postgraduate Physician Assistant Critical Care Residency Program

Methodist Hospital Physician Organization Physician Assistant Residency Program

UMass Memorial Medical Center Physician Assistant Residency Program in Critical Care

Oregon Health and Sciences University

Dermatology

University of Texas Southwestern's Dermatology Physician Assistant Training Program

Emergency Medicine

Albert Einstein Medical Center Physician Assistant Emergency Medicine Residency

Johns Hopkins Bayview Medical Center Emergency Medicine Residency

University of Iowa Emergency Medicine Physician Assistant Residency Program

University of Texas Health Science Center, San Antonio

U.S. Army Medical Department Emergency Medicine Physician Assistant Programs

Wright Patterson Emergency Medicine Physician Assistant Fellowship

Hospitalist

Alderson-Broaddus College

Mayo Clinic Arizona Postgrad PA Fellowship in Hospital Internal Medicine

Neonatology

University of Kentucky PA Residency in Neonatology

Neurosurgery

Geisinger Medical Center Advanced Practice Postgraduate Neuroscience Residency

University of Arizona–Tucson, Neurosurgery PA Residency

OB-GYN

Riverside-Arrowhead Regional Medical Center

Oncology
University of Texas M.D. Anderson Cancer Center Postgraduate PA Residency Program in Oncology

Orthopedic Surgery
Arrowhead Regional Medical Center

Illinois Bone and Joint Institute

Watuga Orthopaedics

Psychiatry
Cherokee Mental Health Institute

Regions Hospital Psychiatry Fellowship for PAs and NPs

Rheumatology
University of Texas Southwestern/Dallas VA Medical Center

Sleep Medicine
Neurology and Neuroradiology Residency Program, Bethlehem, PA

Surgery
Alderson-Broaddus College

Arrowhead Regional Medical Center—General Surgery Physician Assistant Residency

Bassett Healthcare

Duke University Medical Center

Geisinger Medical Center Physician Assistant Surgical Residency Program

Grand Rapids PA Surgical Residency

Hospital of Central Connecticut PA Residency in General Surgery

Johns Hopkins Hospital

Postgraduate Surgical Residency for Physician Assistants

Montefiore Medical Center—University Hospital for Albert Einstein College of Medicine

Norwalk Hospital/Yale University School of Medicine (General)

Mayo Clinic Arizona Postgrad. PA Fellowship in Otolaryngology/ Head and Neck Surgery

Medical College of Wisconsin Post Graduate Physician Assistant Training Program

WakeMed Health and Hospitals PA Residency in Trauma, Critical Care, and General Surgery

Trauma/Critical Care

Bridgeport Hospital PA Trauma, Surgical Critical Care, and Burn Fellowship

Pacific University—Rural Trauma and Hospital Care

St. Luke's Hospital Trauma and Surgical Critical Care

University of Texas Southwestern/Parkland Health and Hospital System Physician Assistant Residency Program in Trauma and Burns

WakeMed Health and Hospitals PA Residency in Trauma, Critical Care, and General Surgery

Urology

Northwest Metropolitan Urology Associates Physician Assistant Urology Residency Program

THE EDUCATIONAL EXPERIENCE

Before we get to the issue of master's versus bachelor's programs, let's examine some other aspects of a program that may be just as important to you and your educational experience.

It is important to remember that, as long as you attend an accredited PA program, you are eligible to sit for the national boards. If you pass the boards, you can work as a PA. For some people, that means that a program that prepares you for the boards may be good enough. However, the quality of the individual PA program may be a deciding factor in whether you apply to one school over another. For instance, some programs teach anatomy using cadavers, whereas other programs use plastic models and slides. Some programs are affiliated with a medical school and enjoy the benefits and facilities that go with it, whereas others are located at a four-year college or a community college. Some programs are taught by MD residents and fellows, whereas others are taught by PAs. Finally, tuition for some programs costs more than $20,000, whereas other programs cost a fraction of that amount. Only you can decide what is most important to you in your educational experience.

Master's Degree versus Bachelor's Degree

One of the most frequent questions I get from prospective PA students is, "To work as a PA, does it matter if you have a bachelor's degree versus a master's degree?" The answer used to be a definitive no. However, the trend in PA education is certainly headed toward master's programs. Many people feel that it's time for PA education to reach the graduate level. In 1997, fewer than 8% of PA school graduates had earned a master's degree from their respective programs. By 2008, that number had jumped to 43%. If you are accepted into a program that offers a master's degree and one that doesn't, you may have to give the matter some additional thought. For instance, if you have aspirations to teach or become a faculty member at a PA program, you will more than likely need a master's degree. Keep in mind, though, that master's-degree programs tend to cost much more than those that offer a certificate or a bachelor's degree. If you don't plan to teach or become a faculty member, it might take you a long time to recoup financially. In addition, there are now many programs that offer PAs the opportunity to earn a master's degree online after they graduate from PA school. Some of those programs are fairly inexpensive but provide the same credentials as the more expensive PA programs.

Pass-Fail Rate

More important than which degree or certificate a PA program offers is the program's first-time pass-fail rate on the national boards. **When considering various programs, be sure to inquire about the first-time pass-fail rate on the boards.** I stress *first-time* because many programs may give you the overall pass-fail rate, which might show, for example, that eventually 90% of graduates pass the boards. However, you need to know how many graduates pass the boards the first time. You should also be aware of the fact that, if you fail the boards on the first try, your odds of passing them decrease significantly each time you sit for the exam.

OTHER ISSUES TO CONSIDER

I have already covered some of the main issues to consider when selecting a program. Let's look at some other factors that may influence your decision.

Clinical Rotations

Once you complete your didactic training, you will embark on clinical rotations, in which you will learn and practice your clinical skills. You will learn to take a thorough medical history and complete a comprehensive physical examination on real patients. You will be required to adapt to various teachers and styles and the intricacies of each facility you work in. You will find that as soon as you begin to get comfortable at one site and learn where all the bathrooms and cafeteria are located, it will be time to move on to your next rotation.

Clinical rotations provide you with an opportunity to grow as a clinician. It is important that the schools you consider have well-established clinical rotation sites that provide a rewarding experience for the student. Most schools have mandatory clinical rotations in family practice, internal medicine, surgery, emergency room, pediatrics, obstetrics and gynecology, and psychiatry. In addition, students can pick from a variety of elective rotations. Because you are the one paying for your education, be sure you get the most for your dollar.

Another suggestion when selecting a program is to talk with students in various programs to find out what they like and dislike about their clinical experience. Ask students about the ratio of medical students to PA students on any given rotation. Are PA students given the same opportunities as the medical students, or are they lower on the food chain? Many programs keep a running file on the various rotation sites with written feedback from students after completing the rotation. Ask if you can read some of those comments, as students tend to comment on everything from the quality of the clinical experience to parking and accommodations. This is valuable information and will serve to guide you when it's time for you to select a program and/or rotation sites when you are a student.

Parking and Housing

How will you get to school every day? Can you afford to pay the going rate for rent in the city or town where you will attend school? You must consider such issues before you decide on any given program. Take into account the cost of living, parking, food, utilities, and so on. A good place to start your research is with the local chamber of commerce, which can mail you enough literature to make an informed decision.

MORE TIPS

The following is a short list of tips that may aid you in the decision-making process. If you follow all of these suggestions, you will be a well-informed applicant. And applicants who do their homework tend to perform well at the interview!

Order the PA Programs Directory

The PA School Programs Directory is offered exclusively by the Physician Assistant Education Association (PAEA). The directory lists all of the accredited PA programs in the United States. It also includes information on tuition, prerequisites, financial aid, tests scores, essay requirements and content, curriculum, and clinical rotations. **The directory is no longer published in a book format but it can be accessed online through the APAP at http://www.paeaonline.org/index.php?ht=d/ContentDir/pid/255.**

Attend the Open House

Attending a program's open house is a must if you are serious about the program. First of all, it gives the program an opportunity to match your face with your name. Most programs also keep a record of open-house attendees, which may eventually help your overall score on your application.

Next, attending the open house gives you insight into the program. By listening to the program speakers you can get a good feel for the philosophy of the program, which can be helpful when writing your essay or interviewing. You also have the opportunity to meet some of the current students and faculty. You might even chat with someone who will interview you later. Of course, attending the open house doesn't guarantee you an interview, but in the highly competitive applications environment, it certainly won't hurt your chances either.

By attending an open house, you also have the opportunity to meet and size up the competition. By speaking with other applicants, especially those who may have interviewed elsewhere, you may get some ideas on ways to strengthen your application. Take this opportunity to soak up as much information as you can from everyone you meet that day.

Finally, after attending the open house you might decide that a particular school is not a good fit for you. Perhaps you are not impressed with the faculty or the quality of the students. Maybe the program appears to be unorganized, which is not uncommon with newer programs. In any case, it is better that you find this out as soon as possible, before you accept a position in a particular class.

Speak with the Program Director

Whether or not you attend the open house, speak to the school's program director at least once before you apply. If you live nearby or plan to visit the area, set up a face-to-face appointment. Again, this is an opportunity to allow someone on the admissions committee to place a face with your name. If you do get an interview with the program director, be sure to dress appropriately and have a list of relevant questions prepared prior to the meeting. Remember, each encounter that you have with program faculty is evaluated in one way or another, so be sure your encounter is a positive one.

Visit Local Hospitals or Clinics

Stop by the local hospital or clinic and see how many of the program's graduates are employed there. Ask the physicians and nurses how they feel about the PAs who work there, and especially the graduates of the program you are interested in. Does the PA school have a good reputation in the community? While you visit the facility, speak to some of the graduate PAs who work there and ask them whether they are happy with the education they received from the program. By the time you leave, you will have a good idea as to the quality of the program.

[CHAPTER 5]

Completing the Application

So now you are ready to take the leap to apply to a PA program. In this chapter, I discuss the procedures for completing the PA school application. I include all of the components that you must deliver to the admissions committee for it to consider you for an interview. Some schools may require that you fill out two separate applications: one application for the PA program and one for the college or university itself. The latter is usually a formality if you meet all of the requirements of the PA program. I also discuss the application process and how committees score and select candidates for interviews. Moreover, I touch on letters of recommendation, pointing out whom you should obtain letters from, what the letters should say, and how to obtain the perfect letter of reference. Finally, I provide detailed information on the relatively new Central Application Service for Physician Assistants (CASPA).

Most applications require the following items:

- Application fee
- Application form(s)
- Test scores (e.g., SAT/ACT, GRE, AHPAT, TOEFL)
- Transcripts (high school and college)
- Three evaluation (reference) letters
- U.S. Government form DD214 (applicable for veterans)
- Professional certificates
- Narrative statement (essay)

If you are reapplying to a program, you should start with new forms—as if you had never applied before. It is especially important to include a new essay. Hopefully, you will be able to favorably update your previous application and present even more evidence that the committee should select you this time.

Each school has its own requirements for admission. **The key on any application is to pay strict attention to detail,** to complete the forms as soon as possible after you receive them, and to send for your transcripts early enough to meet the various program deadlines. In addition, be sure that you meet the program's prerequisites before you apply or that you are at least enrolled in a prerequisite class at the time of application. Indicate on your application whether you are currently enrolled in a prerequisite class so that the committee knows that you will be a fully qualified candidate by the program start date. Occasionally, a program will waive a particular prerequisite on the basis of your prior experience or circumstances. Always make sure to get any waiver in writing.

A professional application should be typed, unless otherwise instructed, and error free. This means that it should have no spelling errors, typos, and so on. A great way to check your application for spelling errors is to read the entire application backward. This may take some time to do, but the results are well worth it. You'll find that by reading the text backward, spelling errors will pop right out of the page. I also recommend that you have at least one other person read your application for errors and overall content.

Spelling errors can be the kiss of death for an applicant. If you aren't able to pay strict attention to detail on an application, how can the committee trust that you will focus on the details of your patients? Will you also miss a critical lab value or a fracture on a child's x-ray? The point is clear: your application can speak volumes about you before the committee even gets to meet you.

THE APPLICATION PROCESS

The typical PA program is approximately two years in length, full-time. A few programs are three or four years in length. Application deadlines vary for each program; however, a general rule is that applications are due between September and January for classes that enter the following summer or fall. If you are applying to a program with rolling admissions, you can submit your application at any time; however, if you do not apply early enough, you may be rolled over until the next year, as it's first come, first served at such schools. Most programs interview students in January and February, so give the committee plenty of time to give your application a fair evaluation.

The application review process is complex, yet comprehensive. The process includes an extensive set of checks and balances to ensure that the best candidates are interviewed. Several committee members may be involved in each application, so no single person controls your fate. Let's take a look at the process and see how successful candidates navigate their way through the system. Keep in mind that the following procedure is from a typical program; each school may evaluate its applicants however it wishes.

Initially, once you have completed the application and submitted all of the supporting material, the program registrar checks your file for completeness, organizes the file, and passes it on for admissions committee review.

Most programs have several volunteers who sit on the admissions committee, evaluate applications, and conduct applicant interviews. The committee comprises program faculty, program PA students, graduate PAs who work in the community, and various other medical professionals.

Each committee member is issued a stack of applications to review and score. That same stack of applications is then passed on to two other committee members for review and scoring. Usually, both male and female committee members review the records. In giving you a score, committee members consider your medical experience, narrative statement (essay), references, work history, and your understanding of the PA **profession. There is no particular factor that influences your overall score more than any other; however, a poorly written essay or a less-than-desirable letter of recommendation can certainly ruin your chances of being invited to an interview.**

Once all of the applicants receive a score, the committee meets to select a group of applicants to interview. The number of applicants who are invited to interview varies from program to program. Many schools, however, interview approximately 100 applicants per year.

Selecting those 100 candidates for an interview involves one final process. After tallying the scores of each candidate, the committee usually unanimously agrees on 75 or so applicants who are clearly and objectively the cream of the crop. It is the selection of the remaining 25 applicants that makes the interview selection process so interesting and sometimes controversial. One committee member may make a very strong case for a particular candidate, whereas 2 other members may argue strongly against that same applicant. Sometimes a spelling error or a poor letter of reference can be the difference between getting accepted and getting rejected.

After the smoke clears and the final cut is made, many committee members ponder over those applicants who were turned down because of spelling errors or a poorly written essay. As a committee member, you always wonder whether you've made the right choices or perhaps let a great prospect slip through the cracks.

In any event, as an applicant, make sure that your application is error free and your essay is well written. This way, you're sure to be evaluated on your strengths rather than your weaknesses.

LETTERS OF RECOMMENDATION

As part of the application process, you are required to provide at least three letters of recommendation in support of your application. Be sure to pay strict attention to detail about each school's specific requirements for references. For instance, some schools may allow you to choose your own personal references. Other programs specify that you should have letters from a PA, a physician, and a former supervisor.

When you are considering potential candidates to provide you with a great letter of reference, be sure to include at least one PA. After all, you are applying to a PA program, and the committee would like to know that you've impressed another PA significantly enough to support your application. The PA profession is relatively small, and most of us (PAs) would not cosign a potential student's application if they didn't think that he or she would make a great PA. To some, this rule is quite obvious; however, plenty of applicants fail to grasp this simple concept. Applicants write about shadowing or working with PAs in their essay but then fail to obtain a reference from such a valuable resource.

Many applicants are under the false impression that the bigger the name or position of a person, the more weight his or her letter of reference will carry. Nothing could be further from the truth. The admissions committee includes some pretty sharp people, most of whom are PAs. The committee will favor a letter from a fellow PA over some big shot on any given day. If you don't know any PAs, don't fret. Get busy locating some local PAs and ask to shadow them for a day or two. Most PAs will jump at the chance to help you.

Your references will usually be asked to rate you in the following areas:

- Academic performance
- Interpersonal skills

- Maturity
- Adaptability and flexibility
- Motivation for a career as a PA

In addition, your references will be asked to provide written comments on the following:

- Applicant's ability to relate well with others
- Strengths relative to a career as a PA
- Weaknesses
- Other comments bearing on the individual applicant

Keep in mind that a good letter of recommendation has four important features:

1. **It shows that the writer truly knows the individual and can comment about the applicant's qualifications.**
2. **It shows that the writer knows enough about the applicant and can make comparative judgments about the applicant's intellectual, academic, and professional abilities in relation to others in a similar role.**
3. **It provides supporting details to make the statement believable.**
4. **It is short, yet concise and sincere.**

When it comes to obtaining great letters of recommendation, there's a valuable lesson to be learned from those in the military. Both enlisted and officer personnel write their own evaluations and simply present them to their supervisors for approval and signature. You can try this with your references as well. This is a great way to ensure that your letters meet all four criteria. If a supervisor (i.e., your reviewer) does not agree with any of your comments, he or she can make changes—but that usually doesn't happen. If you are concerned that your referee is too busy to do an effective job, or maybe doesn't have the best writing skills, you can write the letter of recommendation and simply present it to him or her for evaluation and signature. (See Appendix B for sample letters of recommendation.)

Finally, follow up with your references to be sure that they are aware of any deadlines that need to be met. Be tactful, yet assertive. Remember, this is your future at stake here, and you don't want to be rejected because of a missed letter of recommendation. This is another reason you may want to avoid the a letter of recommendation from a big shot. It can be very difficult to follow up with such individuals: they may simply be too busy to do a timely, effective job for you.

In summary, the letter of reference plays a key role in the evaluation of your application. I encourage you, again, to obtain at least one letter of recommendation from a physician assistant. If you absolutely cannot obtain a PA reference, ask someone who knows you well and can honestly and enthusiastically support your desire to become a PA.

CENTRAL APPLICATION SERVICE FOR PHYSICIAN ASSISTANTS (CASPA)

The PAEA's Central Application Service for Physician Assistants (CASPA) provides a simplified process for applying to physician assistant (PA) programs. Applicants complete one application and submit it online with corresponding materials to the centralized service. Then, CASPA verifies the application components for accuracy, calculates the applicant's grade point average, and sends the materials to the PA programs that the applicant designates. The list of participating PA programs can be found in the "Participating Programs" section of the CASPA Web site (http://www. caspaonline.org).

The CASPA process is a convenient and efficient way to apply to multiple PA programs using a single Web-based application. Participating programs represent the majority of today's accredited PA programs. Applicants receive from CASPA a comprehensive online checklist and instructions to help them more easily navigate the application process. For those applying to more than one program, CASPA reduces or eliminates the need for duplicate application data, letters of reference, test scores (except for GRE or MCAT scores, which the applicant must send directly to the designated programs), and transcripts. Moreover, CASPA provides a real-time applicant portal so that applicants can check the status of their CASPA application, transcripts, and letters of reference online at any time. In addition, CASPA allows applicants to access the application from any computer with Internet access and a standard browser. Applicants can close and reopen their application as often as desired before they submit it.

The CASPA application cycle runs from mid-April to mid-March of each year. Applicants should check the prerequisites and deadlines for the programs to which they wish to apply. Applicants should read the "Before

Applying" section of the CASPA Web site before they begin the application process. Submitting application materials early will ensure timely processing and help avoid delays. Once an application is considered complete, it can take 4 to 5 weeks to process and mail it to the applicant's designated programs.

The application is considered complete when CASPA has received all of the following:

- Electronic application
- All official transcripts
- At least two letters of recommendation
- Payment

Customer support by phone is available for CASPA Monday through Friday from 9:00 AM to 5:00 PM. Eastern Time. In addition to the customer support staff, participating programs can access real-time applicant information via the CASPA Admissions Portal.

CASPA
P.O. Box 9108
Watertown, MA 02471

Helpdesk: CASPA Applicants: (617) 612-2080
Fax: (617) 612-2081
Web: www.caspaonline.org
E-mail: caspainfo@caspaonline.org

For Express/Overnight shipments only*
CASPA
C/O Liaison International
311 Arsenal Street, Suite 15
Watertown MA 02472

Table 5.1 shows the 2009 application deadlines for a variety of CASPA-participating programs (from the CASPA Web site) to give you an idea of the admissions schedule. Please note that these application deadlines can change, so, to protect yourself, make sure you keep up with the current data on the CASPA Web site. The web address is: http://portal.caspaonline.org/faq/ins_programs.htm

Table 5.1. Deadlines for CASPA-Participating PA Programs

State	Program	Program Deadline
AL	University of Alabama at Birmingham	9/1/2009
AL	University of South Alabama	11/1/2009
AR	Harding University	11/1/2009
AZ	A. T. Still University, Arizona School of Health Sciences	11/1/2009
AZ	A. T. Still University, Arizona School of Health Sciences—Native American PA Track	11/1/2009
AZ	Midwestern University Glendale	10/1/2009
CA	Charles Drew University	1/15/2010
CA	Loma Linda University	11/1/2009
CA	Samuel Merritt University	10/1/2009
CA	Touro University—CA Joint MSPAS/MPH Program	11/1/2009
CA	University of California, Davis	10/1/2009
CA	University of Southern California	12/1/2009
CA	Western University of Health Science	11/1/2009
CO	Red Rocks Community College	9/1/2009
CO	University of Colorado Denver	10/1/2009
CT	Quinnipiac University	10/1/2009
CT	Yale University	9/1/2009
DC	George Washington University, 3-year PA/MPH program	10/1/2009
DC	George Washington University, traditional 2-year PA program	10/1/2009
DC	Howard University	1/15/2010

(Continued)

Table 5.1. Deadlines for CASPA-Participating PA Programs (*Continued*)

State	Program	Program Deadline
DE	Arcadia University, Christiana Delaware, 3-Year Dual Masters, PA/MPH	1/15/2010
DE	Arcadia University, Christiana Delaware, 2-Year PA Program	1/15/2010
FL	Barry University, Miami Shores campus	12/1/2009
FL	Barry University, St. Petersburg Campus (Satellite)	12/1/2009
FL	Keiser University, Ft. Lauderdale	12/1/2009
FL	Nova Southeastern University, Ft. Lauderdale	12/1/2009
FL	Nova Southeastern University, Orlando	1/15/2010
FL	Nova Southeastern University, Jacksonville	3/1/2010
FL	Nova Southeastern University, Southwest Florida, Ft. Myers	3/1/2010
FL	South University, Tampa	12/1/2009
FL	University of Florida	10/1/2009
GA	Emory University	10/1/2009
GA	Mercer University (January 2010 start date)	8/1/2009
GA	Mercer University (January 2011 start date)	3/1/2010
GA	South University (January 2010 start date)	9/1/2010
GA	South University (January 2011 start date)	3/1/2010
IA	Des Moines University	12/1/2009
IA	University of Iowa	11/1/2009
ID	Idaho State University	12/1/2009
IL	John H. Stroger Jr. Hospital of Cook County/Malcolm X College	3/1/2010

(*Continued*)

Table 5.1. Deadlines for CASPA-Participating PA Programs (*Continued*)

State	Program	Program Deadline
IL	John H. Stroger Jr. Hospital of Cook County/Malcolm X College	3/1/2010
IL	Midwestern University, Downers Grove	10/1/2009
IL	Rosalind Franklin University of Medicine and Science	12/1/2009
IL	Southern Illinois University, Carbondale	10/1/2009
IN	Butler University	12/1/2009
IN	University of Saint Francis, Indiana	12/1/2009
KS	Wichita State University	10/1/2009
KY	University of Kentucky, Lexington	6/15/2009
KY	University of Kentucky, Morehead	6/15/2009
MA	Massachusetts College of Pharmacy and Health Sciences, Boston	11/1/2009
MA	Massachusetts College of Pharmacy and Health Sciences, Worcester (January 2010 start date)	10/1/2009
MA	Massachusetts College of Pharmacy and Health Sciences, Worcester (January 2011 start date)	3/1/2010
MA	Northeastern University	9/1/2009
MD	Anne Arundel Community College	9/1/2009
MD	Towson University, CCBC ESSEX	9/1/2009
ME	University of New England	10/1/2009
MI	Central Michigan University	10/1/2009
MI	University of Detroit Mercy	1/15/2010
MI	Wayne State University	9/1/2009

(*Continued*)

Table 5.1. Deadlines for CASPA-Participating PA Programs (*Continued*)

State	Program	Program Deadline
MI	Western Michigan University	12/1/2009
MN	Augsburg College	9/1/2009
MO	Missouri State University	8/1/2009
MO	Saint Louis University	12/1/2009
MT	Rocky Mountain College	10/1/2009
NC	Duke University	10/1/2009
NC	East Carolina University	10/1/2009
NC	Methodist University	3/1/2010
NC	Wake Forest University	10/1/2009
NC	Wingate University	1/15/2010
ND	University of North Dakota	9/1/2009
NE	Union College	11/1/2009
NE	University of Nebraska Medical Center	10/1/2009
NH	Massachusetts College of Pharmacy and Health Sciences, Manchester (January 2010 start date)	10/1/2009
NH	Massachusetts College of Pharmacy and Health Sciences, Manchester (January 2011 start date)	3/1/2010
NJ	University of Medicine and Dentistry of New Jersey	10/1/2009
NM	University of New Mexico	9/1/2009
NM	University of St. Francis	12/1/2009
NV	Touro University, Nevada	3/1/2010
NY	Albany Medical College (January 2010 start date)	10/1/2009

(*Continued*)

Table 5.1. Deadlines for CASPA-Participating PA Programs (*Continued*)

State	Program	Program Deadline
NY	Albany Medical College (January 2011 start date)	3/1/2010
NY	Cornell University, Weill Cornell Graduate School, Master of Science in Health Sciences for Physician Assistants Program	10/1/2009
NY	Daemen College	12/1/2009
NY	Hofstra University	3/1/2010
NY	Le Moyne College	10/1/2009
NY	Long Island University	1/15/2010
NY	Mercy College Graduate Program	12/1/2009
NY	New York Institute of Technology	1/15/2010
NY	Pace University, Lenox Hill Hospital	10/1/2009
NY	St. John's University	11/1/2009
NY	Stony Brook University	12/1/2009
NY	SUNY Upstate Medical University	3/1/2010
NY	Touro College School of Health Science, Bay Shore (BS and BS/MS program)	3/1/2010
NY	Touro College School of Health Science, Winthrop Extension Center (BS/MS program only)	9/1/2009
OH	Cuyahoga Community College	11/1/2009
OH	Kettering College of Medical Arts	10/1/2009
OH	Marietta College	11/1/2009
OH	Mount Union College	10/1/2009
OH	University of Findlay, master's-degree program	10/1/2009

(*Continued*)

Table 5.1. Deadlines for CASPA-Participating PA Programs (*Continued*)

State	Program	Program Deadline
OH	University of Toledo	10/1/2009
OR	Oregon Health and Science University	11/1/2009
OR	Pacific University	10/1/2009
PA	Arcadia University, Glenside, 3-Year Dual Master's, PA/MPH	1/15/2010
PA	Arcadia University, Glenside, 2-Year PA Program	1/15/2010
PA	Chatham University	10/1/2009
PA	DeSales University	1/15/2010
PA	Drexel University, Hahnemann	10/1/2009
PA	King's College	12/1/2009
PA	Lock Haven University of Pennsylvania	11/1/2009
PA	Marywood University	12/1/2009
PA	Philadelphia College of Osteopathic Medicine	12/1/2009
PA	Philadelphia University	10/1/2009
PA	Saint Francis University	11/1/2009
PA	Salus University (August 2009 start date)	6/15/2009
PA	Salus University (August 2010 start date)	3/1/2010
PA	Seton Hall University	3/1/2010
SD	University of South Dakota	10/1/2009
TN	Bethel University	10/1/2009
TN	Lincoln Memorial University, DeBusk College of Osteopathic Medicine	11/1/2009
TN	South College in Knoxville	3/1/2010

(*Continued*)

Table 5.1. Deadlines for CASPA-Participating PA Programs (*Continued*)

State	Program	Program Deadline
TN	Trevecca Nazarene University	11/1/2009
TX	Baylor College of Medicine	10/1/2009
TX	Texas Tech University Health Science Center	12/1/2009
TX	University of North Texas Health Science Center	11/1/2009
TX	University of Texas, Pan American	12/1/2009
TX	University of Texas Health Science Center, San Antonio	10/1/2009
TX	University of Texas Medical Branch, Galveston	10/1/2009
TX	University of Texas Southwestern Medical Center	10/1/2009
UT	University of Utah	9/1/2009
VA	Eastern Virginia Medical School	3/1/2010
VA	James Madison University	10/1/2009
VA	Jefferson College of Health Sciences	12/1/2009
VA	Shenandoah University	1/15/2010
WA	University of Washington, MEDEX Northwest	10/1/2009
WI	Marquette University	11/1/2009
WI	University of Wisconsin, La Crosse-Gundersen-Mayo	9/1/2009
WI	University of Wisconsin, Madison	10/1/2009
WV	Alderson-Broaddus College	1/15/2010

[CHAPTER 6]

The Essay

In this chapter, we cover the part of the application process that makes or breaks so many candidates: the narrative statement or essay. Writing the essay creates a lot of stress among applicants for various reasons. Many applicants fear writing in general, and they know the essay has to be not only persuasive but also grammatically correct to score points with the committee. Some applicants struggle with a topic, especially if one is not provided. Others simply don't know how to use the essay effectively to paint an accurate picture without coming off as too self-centered or arrogant.

I designed this chapter to alleviate some of the stress associated with writing your essay. I start by providing you with some suggestions on how to strengthen your essay and how to avoid some common pitfalls. I then give you five specific topics to write about, along with specific instructions for each one of them. Next, I take you through the evolution of an essay to show you how to develop a theme and stick with it. Finally, I provide four complete examples of essays that worked for others, three annotated essays, and some examples from essays that demonstrate persuasive writing techniques.

Before you begin to think about writing your essay, take the time to fill out the worksheets at the end of this chapter. I've included several sheets so that you can gather data on your work history, medical experience, high school and college work, volunteer activities, military experience, foreign-language abilities, travel experiences, and miscellaneous items. By filling out the forms before you start to write your essay, you will have organized your thoughts so that you can write a more effective essay and, in addition, perform better in your interview.

HOW IMPORTANT IS THE ESSAY?

If you were to poll 100 admissions committee members, more than 90% would probably tell you that the essay is the most important part of the application process. Fortunately, the essay is one of the few things over which you have any control. Yes, grade point average, test scores, medical experience, and letters of recommendation are very important, but if you fail to connect with readers of your essay, they may pass over you for an interview. Conversely, otherwise-marginal candidates, with respect to test scores and grade point average, receive interviews strictly on the basis of their very effective, emotionally charged essays.

Serious candidates spend a considerable amount of time writing and rewriting the narrative statement. They have several people read the essay for flow, content, grammar, typos, and spelling. A great technique for catching typos and spelling errors is to read your essay backward; mistakes will jump off the page at you.

The following suggestions will help you write an effective narrative statement. Do not become frustrated if you have trouble finding the exact words at first. The key is to put the pen to the paper and just do it. And remember that under no circumstances is it acceptable to allow someone else to write your essay.

SUGGESTIONS

1. Learn as much as you can about the program you're applying to
If you are going to spend the time, money, and effort applying to a PA program, at least attempt to learn everything you can about the school before you apply or interview. Study the history of the program, including the history of the university or college that offers it. Get a feel for the philosophy of the program and the goals the program sets for educating PA students. Contact as many students and graduates of the program as you can to get a good feel for the strengths and weaknesses of the program. Basically, do your homework, and you'll be a much better and stronger applicant for having done so.

2. Follow instructions
Carefully read the essay questions and be sure your answer is relevant. Too many applicants have their own agenda; they want to tell readers what they want to tell them instead of what the essay asks for. For example, if the essay question is "How do you expect to fulfill your goals as a physician

assistant?" then don't write about your experiences saving lives and volunteering at the soup kitchen. Answer the question!

In addition, if the instructions call for a 2-page narrative, do not write any more than that. In this case, more is not better. Put yourself in the committee members' place: They have already read 50 essays and now come across your 3-pager, with size 8 font, no less. Don't give readers any excuse for not giving it the full attention it deserves.

3. Avoid using first-person *I* too much

To appear less self-centered and more team oriented, read through your essay and limit the number of times you use the word *I*. Instead, use *we, our,* and *us* more often. Give readers the impression that you are a team player. Talk more about your patients than about yourself. **I attended one open house where we were told that if we had more than 5 *Is* in our essay, we should redo them.** This may have been stretching it just a bit, but we certainly got the point.

4. Target your audience

Remember that most committee members are physician assistants. Don't waste a lot of space in your essay writing about the duties and responsibilities of the PA. Believe it or not, many applicants use half of their essay to repeat the AAPA definition of a physician assistant. Use this space instead to tell readers what separates you from the other 10 candidates hoping to get your interview slot.

5. Make it presentable

It goes without saying that you should type your essay on a computer and have it laser printed. If you are instructed to do otherwise, then follow the instructions. Do not type in small fonts; use size 12.

6. Check for spelling

Spelling errors are inexcusable and show a complete lack of attention to detail. The message you are sending to the committee is that you don't care enough about your application, and their program, to give your best effort. This is a sure way to be rejected for an interview. Once you finish your essay, run it through your computer's spell-checker and then have someone you trust read it and provide you with feedback.

7. Organize your writing

Communicating effectively is a key part of the PA's role. If your thoughts are scattered and you cannot organize them, you will have a great deal of difficulty when it comes to explaining procedures to your patients or presenting a patient's symptoms to your attending physician on rounds.

The essay statement is often something like this:

> Attach to this application a typewritten narrative of not more than two pages, explaining where you learned of the PA profession, what factors or influences led you to this career choice, and how you expect to fulfill your goals as a physician associate.

Other programs simply ask you to explain why you want to become a physician assistant. Still other programs may leave the topic up to you (more about this in the next section). Whichever situation applies to you, be sure to read the question carefully and follow the directions.

TOPICS: SELECTION AND DEVELOPMENT

If you have an open-ended essay question, consider writing about one of the following topics:

1. Your motivation for a career as a physician assistant
2. The influences of your family and early experiences on your life
3. The influence of extracurricular or work and volunteer activities on your life
4. Your long-term goals
5. Your personal philosophy

Guidelines

1. Select only those topics about which you have something meaningful to say.
2. Convey your personality in your essay; make yourself appear as an interesting candidate to meet and interview.
3. Add life to your essay. What's important to you? What experiences had an impact on your life? What did you learn as a result of your experiences?
4. Avoid using contractions in an essay. For example, use *did not* instead of *didn't* and *I am* instead of *I'm*.
5. Avoid using abbreviations in your essay unless you have used the complete term first. For example, physician assistant (PA) and emergency room (ER). In general, keep your essay more formal and avoid using abbreviations as much as possible.

6. Avoid slang or colloquial expressions. For example, instead of saying "He is a really cool professor," use "He is a great role model."

7. Avoid using run-on sentences. In other words, keep it simple by avoiding long sentences with excessive punctuation.

8. Make sure your opening paragraph is strong, well constructed, and quickly gains the attention of the reader.

9. Have a key sentence or topic sentence in each paragraph that highlights the main point of the paragraph.

10. Use vignettes, or small anecdotes, as examples to back up what you say. Balance those with explanations.

11. Check the use of tenses and make sure they are consistent.

12. Avoid the use of the passive voice, which is awkward and less effective than the active voice. For example, instead of writing "The job could not be kept because . . .," try "I could not keep the job because . . ."

13. Avoid wordiness.

14. Conclude your essay as strongly as you began it, by reiterating why you want to be a PA (or, for example, what your goals are). A reiteration can add a slightly different slant to what you have already said.

MOTIVATION FOR BECOMING A PA

In the essay, you should address your motivation for a career as a physician assistant. I guarantee you that at some point during the interview, the interviewers will ask you why you want to become a PA. If you discuss this in the essay, you can deal with this question before it is asked and have a helpful outline to work with.

The first thing to do is spend some quiet time thinking about why you want to become a PA. Do some brainstorming. What experiences or people have led you to this career path? Use examples and vignettes to illustrate your point and lend credibility to your essay. The following example illustrates the point:

> Although there were several excellent doctors in our pediatricians' office, we preferred using the physician assistants on our visits. The pediatricians seemed always rushed and spent little time with the physical exam; they were almost mechanical in their mannerisms. The PAs spent much more time with us and developed a special relationship with our children. They knew what sports my

> children were involved in, what grades they received in school, and had an over-all sense of their well-being. Each visit the PA would allow the children to listen to their own heartbeats and always explained every single procedure before she performed it. I later shadowed this same PA and found out that she grew up with a lot of hardship in a rural Southern community. Yet she had a tremendous fol-lowing of patients and enjoyed every minute of her job. I believe a career as a physician assistant will allow me to work autonomously, yet collaboratively, with several members of the health care team. I look forward to the first time I will get to hold a stethoscope up to a child's heart and ask, "Can you hear it?"

Take out a fresh sheet of paper and write this question at the top: Why do I want to become a physician assistant? Start brainstorming and writing down everything that comes to mind—everything goes. If you find that you are having a hard time coming up with the answers, then answer the following questions to try to focus your thoughts:

- Why don't I want to become a physician?
- Why don't I want to become a nurse?
- Why don't I want to become a nurse-practitioner?
- Why don't I want to become a teacher?
- Why don't I want to become a physical therapist?

Hopefully, answering those questions will give you a better understanding of why you want to become a PA. If you are still having difficulty coming up with answers, perhaps you should think hard about choosing this career path.

FAMILY AND EARLY EXPERIENCES

Many applicants feel that they must write about medical experiences or educational awards. **By writing about individuals or incidents that have shaped your life, you begin to paint a picture of an interesting person, someone the admissions committee would like to meet.**

Notice how the following writer uses his childhood experiences to communicate his interest in being a PA:

> I grew up as one of six children. My father died when I was 7, and my mom worked two jobs to support us. She, fortunately, had an education behind her and worked as a nurse in an emergency room. I grew up with plenty of food on the table and a roof over my head, but I had very little guidance. I often got into

trouble and felt lost in life. I did play a lot of sports, though, and as a result, I spent numerous hours in the emergency room where my mom worked. It was there that I became fascinated with medicine. I would peek around corners to watch the doctors perform procedures on patients and beg my mother to let me stay longer. I felt exhilarated in that environment. One day I shared my feelings with one of the residents. He made a statement that I have not forgotten to this day: "Son, you can become anything you want to in life, if you only set your mind to it."

As I grew older, still with no real direction in life, I often thought about those words but never totally bought into the idea. I quit high school at the age of 16 with plans to join the navy when I turned 17. My mother quickly intervened, however, and arranged for me to finish high school during the summer.

That summer, soon after graduation, I enlisted in the navy and became a hospital corpsman. I grew up and matured a great deal in this environment. Most of all, however, I realized why I had such a fascination for medicine. I loved working in the collaborative environment with other health care professionals. I enjoyed providing care to my fellow servicemen and the satisfaction I felt after sewing a marine's leg wound in the field or diagnosing an acute appendix in the clinic. For the first time in my life, I actually enjoyed waking up and going to work in the morning. I looked forward to the challenges that lay ahead. I became eager to learn all that I could and began taking college science courses in the evening. I did very well and began to believe that I could do anything that I set my mind to.

As a result of those experiences, I feel that I have a good understanding of what it takes to provide health care. I understand the role of the physician assistant, and I would like to continue my health care experience and aspirations in this newly expanded role.

EXTRACURRICULAR ACTIVITIES AND WORK AND VOLUNTEER EXPERIENCES

If you have filled out the worksheets at the end of this chapter, writing about extracurricular and work or volunteer experiences should be easy. Keep in mind that you don't always have to write about medical experiences. Show readers what you have learned from all of your life experiences, and try to demonstrate, in your writing, that you are a person of value. Don't simply repeat items (e.g., awards, honors) that you have listed on the application and that readers already know about.

To write effectively, think about answering the following questions in your writing:

- What did you learn from your extracurricular activities or work experiences?
- Are you a team player?
- How have you matured as a result of your experiences?
- If you have held a leadership role, how did you contribute to getting the job done?

The key to success in this area is to lead readers to believe, on their own, that you are an independent thinker and a mature person, without actually using those words in your essay.

The following paragraphs, from two essays, illustrate my point. The writers share what they learned from volunteer and work experiences.

Sample 1

When I decided to volunteer at St. Vincent's hospital, I felt that I had a fairly good idea of how things worked in an emergency room. After all, I had worked as an emergency room technician in one of the largest hospitals in the country. What I did not know, however, was how impersonal and insensitive we can be to our patients. In my role as a patient representative, I came to view things from the other side of the fence: the patient's side. I soon realized that the staff frequently referred to the patients as the leg in room 2 or the belly in room 5. We tell patients, "Your LFTs are elevated" but never stop to explain what LFTs are. We sometimes methodically examine patients and leave them undressed, cold, and embarrassed. We don't ever bother to shut the curtain most of the time.

Because I had some medical experience, I often tried to explain the various procedures to patients and found myself frequently apologizing for the sometimes-insensitive treatment. The patients really appreciated this, and I received numerous letters of gratitude. Soon after starting as a volunteer, I was offered a paid position in patient relations.

As a paid employee, I found myself walking a fine line. I knew that I wanted to become a physician assistant, yet my job was mainly as a patient advocate. As a result, I often had to confront those, who may well have become my future colleagues, with patient complaints that were sometimes aimed at them. I found that if I called patients by their names, instead of by body part, and if I quickly closed a curtain after an exam, that most of the staff started doing the same thing. This provided a much more comfortable environment for the patient and made my job a whole lot easier, too.

Sample 2

Instead of joining the civilian arena after graduating from college, I decided to join the U.S. Air Force. I entered Officer Training School not knowing what to expect but with a lot of expectations. This service paid off in many ways. First, I learned to pay strict attention to detail. Second, the responsibility I had as a junior officer gave me the confidence to perform and accomplish many tasks working under less-than-ideal situations. Third, I learned the importance of teamwork and how to delegate responsibility to get a job done. Finally, I learned to always give 100% because many people relied on me and trusted my judgment. I left the air force with many accomplishments, including the Junior Officer of the Year award.

If you are a volunteer or working as a technician in the health care field, be careful not to profess that you know what it is like to be a physician assistant. However, try to let readers know that you have thoroughly investigated the field and that you can write an intelligent and interesting essay.

IRREGULARITIES IN YOUR ACADEMIC RECORD

Most programs require you to send a copy of your college and high school transcripts with your application. Many people have excellent academic backgrounds. Many people also have good academic backgrounds. Some applicants, however, have a transcript that contains a few Ds, Fs, or Ws. If that is you, then you must address those grades somewhere on the application form. Some choose to use the essay itself; others use the "Additional Comments" section. Choose whichever you prefer, but if you don't address the issue, you may never get to the interview phase.

If you have many irregularities on your transcript, consider retaking the classes in which you did poorly. When you write about those irregularities, do not make excuses. Offer an explanation as best you can without sounding as if you are a victim of circumstance. Point out that you are aware of the deficiencies in your record and tell readers what you have done about it. What have you learned as a result of your mistakes?

The following applicant explained why he was suspended from school in his freshman year:

> I was accepted to Weaver College on a baseball scholarship. At the time, I was used to being a star athlete and having everything done for me. In my freshman year, I paid more attention to playing baseball and trying to fit in with the team than I did to my studies. As a result, my grades suffered, and I was suspended for the rest of the semester. That gave me a lot of time to think about which direction I was headed in. Yes, I came to college to play baseball, but my goal was to get a good education so that I could someday fulfill my dream of working in health care. On returning to school that next semester, I promised myself that I would change my ways and give my education top priority. I worked hard and have maintained a solid 3.3 grade point average since then. I also learned that it does not have to be all or nothing, as I continued playing baseball and volunteering at the local hospital.

The following is an example of a poor explanation for below-average grades. The writer assumes no responsibility for her part in the deficiencies and the paragraph reflects negatively on her as a mature, responsible candidate. She is what I call an excusiologist:

> I would like to use this section of my application to write about some of the low grades I have received. I strongly feel that my transcripts do not provide an adequate representation of my ability to perform well as a physician assistant student. For example, in my sophomore year, I took organic chemistry with the same instructor for two semesters and received Ds both times. The professor and I did not hit it off very well, and I feel that he held this against me when scoring tests and lab assignments. With regards to the F in psychology, my entire grade was based on a paper that we had to hand in at the end of the course. My paper was two days late because I was away taking care of my mother, who was suffering from a serious heart illness. I notified the instructor before I left that my paper might be late. I assumed that it would be all right, but when I received my grade, it was too late to do anything about it. I spoke with my guidance counselor, but he informed me that the syllabus clearly stated that the final paper must have been handed in on time to receive a passing grade; there was nothing he could do. My attempts to contact my instructor and talk it over with her were also futile and the grade stands.
>
> As far as the rest of the low grades are concerned, I feel as though two main factors contributed to my deficiencies. First of all, I went to a very poor high school. Many of the students were more interested in partying than studying. As a result, the teachers were frustrated and did not do a very good job trying to motivate the class. Once I got to college I had a lot of catching up to do and my grades suffered. In addition, I overloaded myself with science courses and labs in my junior year because I switched majors. I always had two or three lab

reports to do per week, and this took up a great deal of time that I would ordinarily have spent studying. In my senior year, however, I really settled down and achieved a 3.5 average for the year.

This explanation is too lengthy and full of excuses. Readers of this essay are likely to put it to one side and go on to a more interesting candidate.

NONTRADITIONAL BACKGROUND

Applicants may be nontraditional by virtue of a number of factors: age, cultural background, medical experience, academic background, GPA, or life experience. Too many applicants feel that they are at a disadvantage because of these factors. In reality, however, a student from a nontraditional background is sometimes a more interesting candidate than the traditional applicant. It all depends on how you present yourself, and your story, to the reader. You must learn to turn your own particular situation into a positive experience.

The following excerpt is from a young woman who explains how her degree in dance and her work in massage therapy qualify her as a strong candidate:

> Through my degree in dance and kinesiology, I learned of the many intricate movements the human body is able to perform, as well as the limitations of muscles, bones, and joints. Soon after graduating, I opened a small practice as a massage therapist. I worked with a variety of patients and found that my best skill was listening intently to complaints and spending enough time with the patient to work those complaints out. I continued to study anatomy and physiology to best serve my patients. I now have a longing to do more. I would like to build on what I have learned and begin to diagnose and treat patients in the medical arena. I am confident that my prior experience will aid me in this quest.

That applicant also does a great job demonstrating that she possesses transferable skills. Although she has not worked directly in a clinical setting, she does a good job of telling readers that the skills she has learned as a massage therapist will suit her well as a physician assistant.

LONG-TERM GOALS

In the essay or interview, you may be asked to comment on your future plans. It may be unrealistic for applicants to know exactly what they want to do when they finish school. If you do have some definite plans, however, and something substantial to say, then by all means mention them. But if you have no definitive plans, then tell the committee that you are exploring several options and wish to keep an open mind at this time. Once you finish your clinical training, you may have a better idea.

PERSONAL PHILOSOPHY

Writing about personal philosophy can be a very dangerous essay area. We all have our own convictions about certain topics, but it is always best to express them conservatively or to show both sides of an issue. If you can speak intelligently and maturely about a topic that may give readers some more insight into you as a person, then you can speak on that subject. But avoid controversy at all costs. The last thing you want to do is get involved in a controversy.

REAPPLICANTS

People applying again after having been rejected previously should write a completely new essay. Be sure to mention how you have grown and what you have learned since the previous year. Also, send in fresh letters of reference along with your application. You must show that you have made some positive changes since your last application.

When you sit down to write your second essay, other issues and concerns may arise. I recommend that you think about the following:

- Your initial thoughts after receiving your letter of rejection.
- How you felt and reacted after the disappointment wore off.
- Did you call the director of the program (after the interview) and ask why you were not accepted?
- Your reaction to the director's comments and your subsequent behavior.
- What have you done since speaking with the program director?
- Have you made any progress since your last application?
- Have you had any significant changes in grades or work experiences?
- Why are you now a better candidate than last year?

Now, it is time to rewrite your essay from a reapplicant's point of view. Focus on the last question: **Why are you now a better candidate than last year?**

EVOLUTION OF AN ESSAY

The following essay is a first draft from a young woman applying to a PA school. After presenting the draft, I'll dissect it by paragraph and rewrite it so it is more effective:

> When I was young; I vividly remember dressing up as a doctor for Halloween and dreaming of becoming one "When I grew up." At that early age, I viewed those in the health professions through rose-colored glasses, as though I thought they could heroically heal people through an injection or a prescription. However, during a hospital internship my senior year, in high school, I realized that the OR is not always that miraculous center of recovery I had once envisioned. While observing a craniotomy, I watched a patient die on the operating table. I was shocked at the emotional distance the health care team showed, then realized death was something inevitable that health care providers face everyday. The physicians, along with the rest of the health care team fulfilled their obligation; to try to cure the patient of a malignant brain tumor. It was then I learned that although modern medicine can prolong life, in the long run, it is death that wins because of the limitations of the human body. However, I decided that merely observing death impassively was beyond me, that I would wish to interact with the patients more intimately than the physician can.
>
> After graduating high school, for two consecutive summers I interned for an orthopedic surgeon. Although I had seen PA's previously, the first time I really took note of one was outside the OR watching her comfort a patient just about to enter the OR. She was explaining exactly what was going to happen once the patient would enter the OR. I could tell that the patient deeply appreciated this extra attention he wouldn't have otherwise received. Later, while reviewing the patient's chart prior to his surgery, I struck up a conversation with an orthopedic PA. As we chatted outside the OR, she asked me whether I planned to go to medical school. Though I had always known I wanted to work in the health care field, I was not sure that I really wanted to become a physician. The aspect of diagnosing and treating patients was what I wanted to do. However, I did not want to spend the next ten to twelve years of my life in school, nor did I seek the confinement and lack of family time a doctor experiences. As my new friend described her profession, I could discern her enthusiasm for it and her caring personality, both of which struck a responsive chord

within me. Until I met this PA, I was unaware of how my character and the traits requisite for being a PA coincide.

Every chance I received, I took advantage of my opportunities to investigate the functions of a PA. More and more I became interested in the PA's ability not only to make decisions autonomously but to work as a team with other physicians and nurses. I relish the notion of interacting directly with my patients and help select the optimal way to comfort and cure them. I was also struck by the PA program's versatility and flexibility, which allow me to change specialties if I desire. Being an independent thinker, as well as a people oriented individual, I have concluded that I am well suited not just for the medical field but for a lifetime career as a PA.

I look forward to this fall to furthering my experience with PA's, when I will be shadowing a PA in the ER of Austin's Brackenridge Hospital. I know that further acquaintance with this position will enhance my understanding of what, I hope, my life's career and help prepare me for its rigors and rewards. Nevertheless, I am already positive that I have found my true calling in life and eagerly anticipate working together with my PA colleagues assisting others to return to the sometimes rock-strewn road to good health. Because the operating room has always been my passion, I most likely will want to concentrate in that area, but as a highly receptive and open-minded person, I will be more than willing to change and focus in different spheres of health care if the occasion to do so arises.

In essence, my background in the medical field and witnessing many different procedures have convinced me that my lifetime dream can best come to reality through dedicating myself to a career as a PA.

Paragraph 1.

This writer uses word pictures to try to make her essay more interesting. The problem is that her sentences are sometimes awkward and confuse the reader. She also, unintentionally, makes it sound as though the health care team is cold and uncaring instead of professional and objective. In addition, she uses abbreviations without first using the complete term. Finally, she speaks of death as being in competition with life; death is a part of life.

Paragraph 2.

The opening sentence is awkward. She uses *PA's* instead of *PAs*. She assumes that the patient would not have received the proper attention were it not for the PA. She uses the colloquial word *chatted*. She writes "nor did I seek the confinement and lack of family time a doctor experiences." This sentence is awkward and an admissions committee is not interested in what someone did not seek.

Paragraph 3.
In the first sentence, the writer needs to explain when and where she took advantage of her opportunities to investigate the functions of PAs. She also has a big problem with tense. Because she is describing how she wants to become a PA, she should be writing either in the conditional tense or the future tense, stating, "I was also struck by the PA program's versatility and flexibility, which will allow me to change specialties if I desire."

Paragraph 4.
This paragraph has numerous spelling and grammatical errors. She uses the awkward phrase *rock strewn*. She also becomes a little too self-centered: "as a highly receptive and open-minded person."

Paragraph 5.
This paragraph needs to be grammatically stronger without the participle *witnessing*.

Here is the final version of the same essay:

> When I was a child, I vividly remember dressing up as a doctor for Halloween. At that early age, I viewed those in the health profession through rose-colored glasses, as if they could heroically heal people through an injection or with a prescription. However, during a hospital internship in high school, I realized that the operating room (OR) is not always the miraculous center of recovery that I had envisaged. While observing a craniotomy, I watched a patient die on the operating table. I was shocked that the health care team seemed to handle this with considerable objectivity and emotional distance, until I realized that death was an inevitability that health care providers face every day. The physicians and other members of the health care team had fulfilled their obligation: to try to cure the patient of a malignant brain tumor. I learned that, although modern medicine can prolong life, in the long run, death is unavoidable because of the limitations of the human body. However, I decided that merely observing death impassively was beyond me and that I wanted to interact with patients more closely than a physician has the time to do.
>
> After graduating from high school, I interned for an orthopedic surgeon for two consecutive summers. Although I had seen PAs previously, the first time I really took note of one was outside the OR, where I watched her comfort a patient about to undergo a surgical procedure. The PA explained exactly what

would happen to him once he entered the room. I could tell that the patient deeply appreciated this extra attention as he began to smile and his face became more relaxed.

Later, while reviewing another patient's chart prior to her surgery, I began speaking with an orthopedic PA, Sherry. As we talked outside the holding area, she asked me whether I planned to go to medical school. Although I always knew I wanted to work in health care, I was not really sure that I wanted to become a physician. On the one hand, I wanted the challenge of diagnosing and treating patients, but on the other hand, I did not want to invest ten years of my life in pursuing that goal. I also have plans to raise a family someday and relish the idea of spending as much time as possible with them. As my new acquaintance described her profession, I could discern her enthusiasm for it and her caring personality, both of which struck a responsive chord in me. Until I met Sherry, I was unaware of how my character and the traits of a good PA coincide.

Every chance I received after that meeting, I took advantage of my opportunities to investigate the functions of PAs working in various fields. More and more, I became interested in the PA's ability not only to make decisions autonomously but also to work collaboratively with other members of the health care team. I look forward to being able to interact directly with my own patients and to, one day, be able to comfort them—and I hope to play a significant role in curing them, too. Being an independent thinker and working in a very versatile and flexible career are all very appealing to me.

This fall, I look forward to furthering my experience with PAs by shadowing a PA in the emergency room of Austin's Brackenridge Hospital. I am confident that my further acquaintance with this position will enhance my understanding of what I hope to be my life's career and help prepare me for its rigors and rewards. Nevertheless, I am positive that I have found my true calling in life, and I eagerly anticipate working together with my PA colleagues to assist others to return to the sometimes-difficult road to good health. Because the operating room is my passion, I will more than likely want to concentrate in surgery, but as a receptive and open-minded person, I will be willing to change and focus in different arenas of health care if the occasion to do so arises.

In essence, my background in the medical field and the fact that I have witnessed PAs working in various environments have convinced me that my lifetime dream can best come to fruition through dedicating myself to a career as a PA.

My other recommendation to this candidate was to provide examples of other skills, collaborative work experiences, and organizational duties or functions.

ESSAYS THAT WORKED

Schools can vary in the length of the essay. I've included samples in this section of 500-word and longer essays. Remember to stick closely to the guidelines recommended by the school to which you are applying.

Sample 1

Attach to this application a typewritten narrative of not more than two pages, explaining where you learned of the PA profession, what factors or influences led you to this career choice, and how you expect to fulfill your goals as a physician assistant.

For four years in the mid-1970s I was a Navy Corpsman, providing direct medical care to more than 400 marines, often in conditions of urgency and with little or no supervision. During this time I was exposed to the drama and trauma associated with medical care on a day-to-day basis. I learned how to work under conditions of limited or imperfect information and how to maintain composure under stress. Most important, I felt firsthand the profound satisfaction that comes from successfully delivering medical care.

After an honorable discharge from the navy in 1979, I worked in the Yale–New Haven Hospital as an emergency room technician. During that time, I had a chance to develop my skills as a team worker in a collaborative environment. This experience significantly broadened my view of disease and death, as the majority of our patients were not healthy young men as they tended to be in the military. I saw the direct effects of disease on infants, children, adolescents, adults, and elderly people of all ages, ethnic backgrounds, and socioeconomic conditions.

At Yale–New Haven, I worked closely with a physician associate. This was the first time I had ever been exposed to this career. His obvious technical expertise and medical knowledge were impressive. However, the profession was far less developed than it is today. I left the emergency room knowing that I wanted to pursue my career interests in health care but unsure of which route to follow. I then decided to earn a four-year degree in chemistry.

During my junior year in college, my career plans were changed drastically by the birth of my first child. Because I did not wish to continue to head a household as the proverbial starving student, I decided upon graduating to rejoin the military, in this case the air force. This represented a degree of security to me for the time being.

For the past several years, I have been an industrial salesperson. It has been quite rewarding in that it has allowed me to provide a good standard of living for myself and my family. However, it does not give me the deep satisfaction I receive from my hospital volunteer work. I have the feeling that anyone could sell the products I sell but that service as a health professional is a genuine honor and calling.

So, what, at my age and professional level, is the best way to become a health professional? To attempt to go to medical school would be an enormous investment of time and money. I have considered nursing or acting as a nurse-practitioner, but I am more interested in the technical and diagnostic aspects of medicine and the close partnership with a physician that being a physician associate can give.

In my deliberations over making this career choice, I have talked extensively with physicians, physician associates, and other health care professionals. I have taken further coursework and done well. One of the reasons that the profession of physician associate appeals to me as a long-term career choice is the opportunity to directly influence people in a positive way. Specifically, I am referring to the importance of continuing to emphasize in a strong but helpful way the basics of preventive medicine. In the past, a relative and two close friends died from preventable diseases. This has dramatically shown me the responsibility a caregiver has in encouraging habits that prolong and improve the quality of life.

I have come to see and believe strongly in the concept that good medicine comes not only from bottles and boxes but also from the heart and feelings of the caregiver. To be truly effective as a physician associate, I will have to excel in technical ability and medical knowledge, and as a communicator. Very few people can, in the course of their work, help save or significantly prolong a life. As a physician associate, I will have the opportunity of taking a minute to talk about why stop smoking or go on a diet. This to me is a true measure of a career satisfaction.

One of the most valuable aspects of my experience has been the opportunity to work with and for outstanding individuals. These people are not only scientifically rigorous with information but also extremely humane in their dealings with others, both colleagues and patients. One such individual is a physician associate with whom I work at St. Raphael's Hospital. She is energetic, positive, personable, and seems to always have a moment and a good word for everybody. Above all, she is a total professional and earns by her daily efforts the respect of those she works with.

The Physician Associate Program is an ideal way to realize career ambitions in health care. Physician associates have the chance to act at a significant level of intervention with patients without needing to invest the years and years of training that becoming a physician would require.

If given the opportunity, I plan to use my physician associate training to return to the emergency room in a newly enhanced role. This, to me, is where so much of the opportunity exists to practice the skills I have and will develop. I enjoy the direct contact with people, the fast-changing environment, and most of all the chance to directly work with and help people who are in serious need.

With the AIDS epidemic, the prevalence of teen violence, and the enormous substance abuse problems today, I am sure that there will be more need than ever for skilled, competent individuals to assist in this critical area.

Now here is the same essay in fewer than 500 words:

As a navy corpsman, I spent four years providing direct medical care to more than 400 marines, often in conditions of urgency and with little or no supervision. I was exposed to the drama and trauma associated with medical care on a day-to-day basis. I learned how to work under conditions of limited or imperfect information and how to maintain composure under stress. Most important, I experienced the profound satisfaction that comes with the ability to successfully deliver medical care to people in need.

After an honorable discharge from the navy, I worked in the Yale–New Haven Hospital as an emergency room technician. This experience allowed me to develop my skills as a team worker in a collaborative environment. It significantly broadened my view of disease and death, as most of our patients were not healthy young men, as they tended to be in the military. I witnessed the direct effects of disease on infants, children, adolescents, adults, and elderly people of all ages, ethnic backgrounds, and socioeconomic conditions.

At Yale–New Haven, I worked closely with a physician associate. This was the first time I had been exposed to the career. I was impressed by the PA's technical expertise and medical knowledge. However, the profession was far less developed then than it is today. I left the emergency room knowing that I wanted to pursue a career in health care but unsure of which route to follow.

I decided to pursue a 4-year degree in chemistry. During my junior year in college, my career plans changed drastically with the birth of my first child. Because I could not head a household as the proverbial starving student, I decided to rejoin the military upon graduation, in this case the air force. That decision provided a degree of security to me for the time being.

I have been an industrial salesperson over the past several years, which has allowed me to provide a good standard of living for myself and my family. However, it does not allow for the deep satisfaction I gain from working directly with patients. I feel that anyone could sell the products I sell but that the service that a health professional provides is a genuine honor and calling.

If given the opportunity, I plan to use my physician associate training to return to the emergency room in a newly enhanced role. This, to me, is where so much of the opportunity exists to practice the skills I have learned and will continue to develop. I enjoy the direct contact with people, the fast-changing environment, and most of all the chance to help and to work directly with people who are in serious need.

Sample 2

Tell the committee what factors led you to choose a career as a physician assistant, and how you have prepared yourself for this role.

My decision to seek a career in medicine was influenced by several personal and work-based experiences. However, it was my grandfather, a very important person in my life, who played a significant role in finalizing my career choice. Shortly after my thirteenth birthday, he was hospitalized with a heart attack. He subsequently underwent heart surgery and suffered a stroke in the immediate postoperative period. I felt overwhelmed by the fact that no one seemed to be able to do anything to help him. One day while I sat at his bedside I realized that I wanted to get involved in medicine, and I promised him that I would work hard to be able to help others get well. The next week he died, and I became more determined than ever to make a difference by caring for others.

Over the past several years, my interest in becoming a physician assistant has been strengthened by my extracurricular and work activities. While in high school I worked as a unit clerk, part-time, on a busy surgical floor. It was there that I was briefly introduced to the work of PAs. My duties consisted of answering the phone, ordering lab tests, and at times interacting with the patients. As a result of that exposure, I became familiar with medical terminology, learned about the health care "team" concept, and played a significant role in recruiting volunteers to our floor to spend time with our patients. During the summer of 1990, I received my first hands-on experience and my first direct contact with PAs. I worked as a technician in the emergency room alongside nurses, doctors, technicians, and PAs. I collected and measured vital signs, obtained short medical histories, assisted in trauma cases, and sometimes just held patients' hand to comfort them. It was there that I learned that the practice of medicine is as much about good caregiving as it is about the appropriate drug therapy.

In 1992, while studying chemistry at Southern University, I participated in numerous extracurricular activities, thus enhancing my leadership and interpersonal skills. These activities provided situations in which I was allowed to exercise my capabilities as president, vice president, treasurer, and secretary. For instance, in my role as president of the Spanish club, I initiated activities such as a winter coat drive for inner-city Hispanic children and worked with a team of community leaders and students to achieve our goal of collecting more than 1,000 coats.

I have also been involved in other activities, which have given me the opportunity to help those who are socioeconomically disadvantaged and unable to care for themselves. This volunteer work ranged from working at the Saint

Ann's soup kitchen and reading to the blind to holding and feeding "crack babies" in the Newborn Intensive Care Unit at Michener Hospital. As a result of those experiences, I learned to reach out to others and help make a positive change in their lives. I also made quite a few new friends along the way. At Michener Hospital, I also worked on the crisis hotline, where my responsibilities were to be an attentive, confident listener and to provide callers with reference information pertinent to their inquiries. Through that experience, I have gained confidence in dealing with crisis situations.

During my senior year at Southern, I was employed by the local veteran's hospital as a cardiac rehabilitation aide. I worked very closely with patients recovering from either bypass surgery or from heart attacks. I walked with patients, counseled them on proper nutrition, and helped develop an exercise regimen for the Take Heart program. This experience improved my ability to listen to patients and to teach them at the same time.

Presently, I am a volunteer with the Orange County Fire Department. I work as an emergency medical technician. The experience is teaching me how to work under extreme conditions of stress.

My desire to become a physician assistant is sincere and founded on a working knowledge of the role of PAs. I am committed to doing whatever is necessary to achieve my goal.

Now here is that same essay in fewer than 500 words:

Shortly after my thirteenth birthday, my grandfather had a heart attack. He subsequently underwent heart surgery and suffered a stroke in the immediate postoperative period. I was overwhelmed that no one seemed to be able to help him. I realized in the days and evenings that I sat by his hospital bed that I wanted to be involved in medicine. I promised him that I would work hard to gain the tools I would need to be an effective health care provider. He died the next week, and I became more determined than ever to achieve this goal.

I was first exposed to the physician assistant profession in high school through my job as a unit clerk on a busy surgical floor. I became familiar with medical terminology, learned about the health care "team" concept, and played a significant role in recruiting volunteers to our floor. During the summer of 1990, I received my first hands-on experience and my first direct contact with PAs. I worked as a technician in the emergency room alongside nurses, doctors, technicians, and PAs. I collected and measured vital signs, obtained short medical histories, assisted in trauma cases, and sometimes just held patients" hands to provide comfort.

While studying chemistry at Southern University, I enhanced my leadership and interpersonal skills by participating in numerous extracurricular activities. As president of the Spanish club, for example, I initiated activities such as a winter coat drive for inner-city Hispanic children and worked with a team of community leaders and students to collect more than 1,000 coats. I have had many other experiences helping people who are socioeconomically disadvantaged and unable to care for themselves. My work has ranged from helping at the Saint Ann's soup kitchen and reading to the blind to holding and feeding "crack babies" in the Newborn Intensive Care Unit at Michener Hospital. I also worked on the hospital's crisis hotline, where I learned to be an attentive, confident listener and to provide callers with reference information pertinent to their inquiry.

During my senior year at Southern, I was a cardiac rehabilitation aide at the local veteran's hospital. I worked closely with patients recovering from either cardiac bypass surgery or from heart attacks. I walked with them, provided counseling on proper nutrition, and helped develop an exercise regimen for the Take Heart program. This experience improved my ability to listen to patients and to educate them at the same time.

I am currently a volunteer emergency medical technician with the Orange County Fire Department. This experience is improving my ability to work under extreme conditions of stress. The experience has been particularly rewarding and has furthered my resolve to pursue a career as a physician assistant.

Sample 3

The following applicant was accepted to every program that she applied to: Duke, Yale, Northeastern, and George Washington. She has a rich cultural and ethnic history, and she uses her experiences very effectively.

The majority of my extracurricular activities fall under the following categories:

A) Music

I began to take flute lessons in 1974 at the age of 7 and at 13 also began violin lessons. I have become quite accomplished on both instruments and have played in various musical ensembles. Presently I play first flute in the Stratford, Connecticut, Community Band, of which I am the youngest member, and first-flute in the Fairfield University Flute Choir, which I helped organize in 1986. From 1981 to 1983, I played first violin in the Bridgeport, Connecticut, Youth Symphony, and the Sherwood Orchestra. Other ensembles include the Fairfield University Chamber Orchestra and groups annually assembled by my music teachers to regularly perform for residents of convalescent homes. Over the years, I have also played in local bands and done solo performances at various private parties and organizational functions.

B) Ethnic Activities

My home life is quite unique in that my parents are immigrants from Czechoslovakia, and as a result I am able to speak, read, and write the Slovak language fluently. I greatly value my Slovak heritage and culture, and thus a great deal of my time is spent on ethnic activities.

From 1986 to 1987, I served as the general chairman of the centennial celebration of the St. John Nepomucene Society, the oldest Slovak fraternal society in New England. My leadership abilities were strengthened by this event, for, having been given a free hand by the society officers, I directed all arrangements and preparations. This yearlong activity culminated in a successful weekend program highlighted by religious services and a banquet attended by more than 360 people.

In August 1988, I was selected to be a delegate to the 32nd National Convention of the First Slovak Wreath of the Free Eagle, a national Slovak American fraternal society that was organized in 1986. At the convention, I was appointed to serve on the bylaws committee and as assistant secretary of the convention. I was also honored by being elected to the office of supreme youth director. I was not only the youngest member in attendance at the convention but also the youngest, in the ninety-two year history of the organization, to be elected to the board of directors.

To conserve and perpetuate our Slovak culture and traditions, the Slovak societies also sponsor weekly radio programs, which I help produce. At WWPT, Westport, Connecticut, I help produce and coordinate the *Slovak Alliance Program*, which presents traditional folk songs from Slovakia. At WSHU, Fairfield, Connecticut, I help produce and coordinate *Music from Slovakia*, which presents both classical and traditional music written or performed by Slovak composers and ensembles.

C) Work Experience

To help finance my education, I work throughout the year. From September 1984 to May 1987, I was a counter worker at a dry-cleaning establishment, averaging 35 hours per week during the school year and 50 hours per week during the summer months. A most enjoyable aspect of this job was the constant contact I had with the public. The interaction with various people certainly sharpened my social skills.

From June 1987 to present, I have worked for a dermatologist and average 25 hours per week. As a medical assistant at the physician's office, I have gotten hands-on experience and insight into how a physician works in a private practice and how a medical office is run. My duties range from reception to assisting the doctor or nurse.

As a receptionist, I log in patients and make them feel comfortable and answer questions regarding medications, services, and surgeries. The clerical aspect includes typing referral letters and reports, billing, and handling health insurance claims. I often assist the doctor with minor surgery, which also includes preparing specimens for the pathology lab and charting. Most interesting has been my observation of and assistance with hair transplantation surgery, microscopic work, and phlebotomy necessary for the Fibrel injections used in scar and wrinkle treatment. At the office I also make up solutions of Minoxidil used in the treatment of hair loss, monitor the blood pressure of Minoxidil patients, and make up a moisturizing cream with Tretinoin (Retin-A) used to prevent skin wrinkles and acne.

In addition, I am presently a teaching assistant for the freshman biology lab at Fairfield University, a volunteer therapist's assistant for a program for handicapped children, and will soon be certified to perform cardiopulmonary resuscitation (CPR). My experiences in the health care field are quite varied and not only have expanded my medical knowledge but also have provided me with valuable practical experience.

D) Miscellaneous

My other community activities include working as a volunteer at the Easter Seals Rehabilitation Center, in Bridgeport, Connecticut, where I work with young children suffering from mental and physical handicaps. I also volunteer my time at the Merton House soup kitchen, Bridgeport, Connecticut, which provides food and clothing for the poor and homeless.

E) Why I Want to Pursue a Career in Medicine

Sometimes a person experiences one significant event that changes her life and outlook. For me it occurred in 1978, when my father suffered a severe skull fracture due to a fall from a ladder. He remained in a coma for 5 days, but luckily, he completely recovered from his injuries. This close encounter with death left me with a greater appreciation of and respect for life. Most important, however, this experience gave me an incentive. I am forever indebted to God and to the physicians for caring for my father's life, and my career choice is my way of repaying this debt. I am willing to make many more sacrifices to achieve my goal, and if I can help others just as my father was helped, and if I can inspire someone just as I was inspired, I know all of my work and sacrifice will not be in vain. This calling comes from deep within me, and I am confident that I can and will achieve my goal.

Sample 4

The focus of the following candidate's essay is on making a career change, as she is an older applicant.

My first exposure to the physician associate profession was in 1983, when a PA at CHCP treated me for a minor medical problem. I asked the universal question

"What is a PA?" and spoke with the PA briefly about his work. Since then, I have had regular contact with PAs through my health insurance providers. Once I seriously considered the PA profession for myself, I read professional journals, the *Physician Assistant Journal* and the *Journal of the American Academy of Physician Assistants*, and talked with PAs to learn more about the profession.

I am currently looking to make a change in my career. The last few years have been a time for reflection and change, with a focus on reviewing my career objectives. I have come to the conclusion that I want to be involved in a career that

- Has a bright future
- Is directly involved with people
- Is in the medical arena
- Meets my need for continuing education and opportunity for change
- Will use my past life and work experiences and skills

The physician associate profession meets all of those criteria.

There is no question as to the viability of the PA profession. Certainly, the creation of a national health care system that demands affordable health care will only increase that need. Indicators predict that the PA profession will be growing for the next decade and beyond. I still have another 20 to 25 years of work ahead of me and want my next profession to be one that will offer a lot of opportunity.

My need to be involved with people has been life long. I have been able to meet this need through volunteer experiences as well as through the evolution of my career. In my first position as a horticulture manager, I worked directly with individuals who have different needs, planning and providing vocational rehabilitation programs. I met with their families and, at times, found myself in situations that were emotional and challenging. As personnel director, I have worked with staff, applicants, and volunteers in areas of hiring, firing, terminal illness, addictions, work-related injuries, and performance issues.

Within this area, I have had to make tough decisions without letting my personal bias interfere. With these previous experiences, I have developed strong interpersonal skills, which will be a substantial asset to me as a PA.

I now find that I want to become involved with people at a more critical level, focusing on their good health and wellness. My original career interests took me in many different directions. I was very interested in physical therapy and the human sciences but also had a strong attraction to horticulture and the plant sciences. My decision to enter the field of horticulture therapy came when I learned that I could combine my two areas of interest. After 5 years of providing hands-on services in a vocational rehabilitation environment, I felt the need to become part of the administrative team and entered graduate school to study organization and management. Now that I have been in administration for 8 years, I find that my interests are pulling me into the medical field again.

As my life progresses, I have observed in myself the need for a profession that offers a diverse array of opportunities. In addition to the diversity of a PA's career options, I find it revitalizing to be in a profession that requires continuing education. The prospect of a career with broad possibilities and education expansion is both attractive and motivational.

Changing my career will only make sense if I can use my past work experiences and skills. It is in this area that I feel I will be able to give the most back to the PA profession. In my 15 years with SARAH, I have developed and implemented both the horticulture and personnel departments from infancy. I now am in the process of implementing yet another new department for SARAH, quality evaluation, for which I will be the director. As the PA profession continues to flourish, there will be a need for people with an administrative and management background such as mine to create and administer the growing number of programs and services that PAs will be providing.

I consider returning to school as an "older" student a very exciting opportunity. The time I spent at Antioch New England Graduate School was one of the most stimulating periods of my life thus far. The experience of working 40 hours per week at SARAH and going to school nights in Hartford and weekends in Keene, New Hampshire, lifted me to a level of energy and motivation that was both stimulating and rewarding. I believe that I will be very successful entering the PA program, with its intensive and rigorous curriculum, given my success at Antioch. I look forward to the challenge with excitement and confidence.

At this point in my life, a career move requires much thought and consideration. After reassessing my career options, I feel that this is the time to make a move. The physician associate profession will bring me back to my original interest in medicine and meet all of my career objectives. By combining my successful educational and work history with my original desire and aptitude in the physical sciences, I am confident that you will find me to be an excellent candidate for your program.

I look forward to having the opportunity to meet with you in an interview for student selection to further discuss my interest in the physician associate program.

Sample 5

The following applicant does a good job of explaining how his life experiences prepared him for a career in medicine:

The first time I can recall meeting a physician assistant was in the emergency room of Martin Army Community Hospital, on Fort Benning, Georgia. I was a private, going through basic infantry training, and happened to be clumsy enough to fall from the top of the 40-foot rope climb on the obstacle course. I knew he was an officer, but he obviously was neither a doctor nor a nurse. He pulled a large piece of wood from under my thumbnail and sent me for some x-rays. He determined that I was not mortally wounded and released me to my unit.

I managed to survive basic training, and eventually I wound up as a paratrooper in the 82nd Airborne Division. Throughout the course of my enlistment, I spent a considerable amount of time with our battalion PA. I learned what he did and what options his profession provided him. By the time I left active duty, the physician assistant profession had become a serious consideration for me.

I have wanted a career in medicine for as long as I can remember. I am sure this is because of my father, and the stories I have heard about him. He learned the intricacies of medicine in school, but he was born with the innate ability to care for and about people.

We lived in a small town, amid a million acres of corn, in rural Illinois. My father practiced from a small office that was actually our converted garage. From that office, he took care of the people in our town, on the surrounding farms, and those in the nearby communities. Less than a month after my brother was born, our father left on a house call from which he never returned. He died that night, leaving his sons a legacy of caring and competency that I hear about to this day. My brother never felt the calling of the medical profession as strongly as I have, so he offered encouragement and support to help me achieve my goals. His encouragement stopped when he was killed shortly after I left the military. His death left me as the only one to follow in my father's footsteps.

My life has prepared me for a career as a physician assistant in many ways. I believe that, like my father, I have an innate ability to care for people. Being a leader in the army instilled a great sense of responsibility in me. I learned how to make decisions under pressure and to recognize the consequences those decisions might have. My work as a medical assistant has given me a better understanding of how the medical team works together to satisfy patient needs. It has exposed me to clinical decision making and the complexities of modern medicine. I have worked with physician assistants in a variety of settings and have come to appreciate how their role fits into the team approach to patient care.

My strongest desire in life is to experience the joys and rigors of a profession in medicine much as my father did. I have the ability and desire to help people, but I need the tools to do this. Becoming a physician assistant will give me the tools I need to take the next step in my career. This is the path I am on, and it is where I can offer the most for those who need help.

Here is the same essay in fewer than 500 words:

As a young private going through infantry training in Fort Benning, Georgia, I fell from the top of a 40-foot rope climb on the obstacle course. My clumsiness landed me in the emergency room of Martin Army Community Hospital, where an officer who was neither a doctor nor a nurse treated me. He pulled a large piece of wood from under my thumbnail and sent me for x-rays. He determined that I was not mortally wounded and released me to my unit. This was my first experience with a physician assistant.

I managed to survive basic training, and eventually I wound up as a paratrooper in the 82nd Airborne Division. Throughout the course of my enlistment, I spent a considerable amount of time with our battalion PA. I learned what he did and what options his profession provided him. By the time I left active duty, the physician assistant profession had become a serious consideration for me.

My interest in medicine was born through the stories I was told about my father. He learned the intricacies of medicine in school, but he was born with the innate ability to care for people. We lived in a small town, amid a million acres of corn, in rural Illinois. My father practiced from a small office that was actually our converted garage. From his office, he took care of the people in our town and on the surrounding farms, as well as those in the nearby communities. Less than a month after my brother was born, our father left on a house call from which he never returned. He died that night, leaving his sons a legacy of caring and competency that I hear about to this day.

My life has prepared me for a career as a physician assistant in many ways. I believe that, like my father, I have an innate ability to care for people. Being a leader in the army instilled a great sense of responsibility in me. I learned how to make decisions under pressure and to recognize the consequences those decisions might have. My work as a medical assistant has given me a better understanding of how the medical team works together to satisfy patient needs. It has exposed me to clinical decision making and the complexities of modern medicine. I have worked with physician assistants in various settings and have come to appreciate how their role fits into the team approach to patient care.

My commitment to becoming a physician assistant is strong. I have the ability and desire to help people, but I need further training and knowledge to allow me to do it. Becoming a physician assistant will give me the tools I need to take the next step in my career. This is the path I have chosen, and the one I believe will provide the greatest sense of fulfillment to me.

Sample 6

This candidate catches readers' attention immediately by talking about nature and Jacques Cousteau, a much more interesting opening than "I've wanted to be a physicians assistant for my entire life":

> The mysteries of nature have always fascinated me. While my boyhood friends admired Batman, I idolized Jacques Cousteau. To me, he represented man's unrelenting desire to explore the unknown while demonstrating a deep respect for the natural order of living things. As a child, I consumed countless books on science and spent hours watching documentaries trying to understand the how and why of all aspects of life. I even set up my own pet shop in our basement that eventually contained 100 tropical fish, ranging from a feisty, red-eyed South American manganese to a 2-foot-long silver arrowana. My innate curiosity continues to evolve and is the foundation of my desire to study medicine.
>
> My interest in the natural world took a personal and painful turn during my sophomore year at Providence College. My father suffered a major heart attack, for which he required quadruple bypass surgery and a 4-week stay in the hospital. His illness redefined my role in the family and I suddenly found myself at its head. I traveled regularly from Providence to New Haven to care for my father and provide support to my mother and siblings. This sudden shift of responsibility was reflected in my poor grades. The fragility of life and the importance of family became clear to me. I matured quickly during this difficult time and my ability to persevere grew stronger.
>
> My work experience in health care began with a summer job as a laboratory assistant in the blood chemistry laboratory of the Hospital of Saint Raphael and progressed the following summer to an operating room aide in the ambulatory surgery unit of Yale–New Haven Hospital. I interacted closely with patients before their surgery and upon their discharge. Their appreciation for my support was extremely rewarding and my experience at Yale–New Haven further motivated me to pursue a career in the health sciences.
>
> After graduating from college, I accepted a position as a research assistant at Yale University School of Medicine, department of ob-gyn. I aided in the completion of a study on the effects of growth factor B1 on myometrial tumors and later had the opportunity to work closely with a physician in patient care. It was then that I gained an appreciation for the trust patients have in their health care provider.
>
> After leaving Yale, I worked as a laboratory assistant in the Department of Molecular Genetics at New York Medical College, where we identified the gene that caused ataxia telangiectasia, a neuromuscular disease that strikes young

children. While I enjoyed my research, I missed personal contact with patients. I spent the past summer shadowing physician assistants in the cardiothoracic unit at the Hospital of Saint Raphael, which solidified my interest in clinical medicine. This experience has clarified my image of a physician assistant's role in health care, and has given me a better understanding of what I hope to achieve in this field.

Sample 7

In this essay, the applicant writes about a commitment to serving the underprivileged. Some programs require service as a part of their program. If you are sincere in your desire to serve this group of people, put it in your essay. Be aware, though, that you should apply to such programs only if your interest is genuine. The committee will know early on if your interest is not real.

My interest in becoming a physician assistant is rooted in the desire to provide quality health care to the underprivileged, a group whose health care needs I have perceived to be acute in the course of my volunteer work. As a social justice coordinator for my parish, I organized volunteer efforts at pediatric clinics and orphanages in Baja, California, as well as the L.A. Mission and Catholic Worker. I also represented the parish in a 10-day, 250-mile walkathon from Santa Barbara to Tijuana to raise money for a child welfare agency. The satisfaction I gain from my career achievements pale in comparison to the gratification I derive from working with the underprivileged. Their acute health care needs prompted my desire to become involved in a professional capacity. My goals led to frustration, however, because medical school was not practical for me and I could not see myself in any other allied health careers. The physician assistant profession is the right fit for me because it will allow me to work in public health at a significant level of medical intervention after completing a program that will be challenging, yet practically suited to my lifestyle.

I was first exposed to the profession of physician assistant when my father had double bypass surgery in 1994 and his postoperative care was managed by his cardiologist's staff PA. Helen explained her role to me and I was impressed with the scope of her responsibilities and sensed that this might be the opportunity I had been seeking. I began shadowing Ted Braunstein, a PA in the emergency department of Mount Sinai Medical Center. I was impressed by his clinical knowledge, compassion, and aptitude for patient education. I was also surprised to see the degree of autonomy given Ted by the attending physicians. My experience in the ER was immensely educational. I assisted Ted by obtaining histories and physicals on Spanish-speaking patients. Soon afterward, I was gloving up to help steady patients as Ted performed suturing or lumbar punctures. The technicians taught me how to draw blood, insert Foley catheters, and take vital measurements. Even after 1,500 hours, I am still amazed at the fascinating array of patients and clinical challenges every shift offers.

If given the opportunity, I plan to use my PA training to work in public health. Ideally, I would like to divide my time between an urban tertiary care facility and a rural clinic. Working in such diverse settings will provide me with a strong clinical foundation and an opportunity for continuing education that will benefit both patient populations. Serving those in serious need will fulfill a lifelong goal and doing so in a PA capacity will allow me to use the analytical, community service, and time management skills that I have acquired in my career thus far. My decision to become a PA is based on a working knowledge of the role, and I am committed to making the necessary sacrifices to achieve this goal.

Sample 8

The following essay has a great attention-getting introduction. Readers immediately wonder how she will tie in her desire to be a physician's assistant:

"In two, bring it up two beats till the end, let's take it home ladies!" I exclaimed while coxing my crew. Adrenaline rushing through me, I realized my teammates and I would make history for the URI Women's Rowing team. After working hard throughout our season, we became Atlantic Ten Conference Champions— the first team in eleven years to break another team's winning streak.

As a coxswain, I served as the liaison between my teammates and coaches, relaying important information and decisions between the two parties. I feel that the physician assistant plays a similar role in the health care system, as an invaluable resource to both the patient and the physician. Becoming a PA will provide me with the opportunity to make meaningful contributions to my patients' health care while allowing a level of personal contact that fulfills me.

Working as a physical therapy aide, I feel a deep satisfaction, as well as a sense of success, in helping patients toward recovery. My experience has taught me that different people respond to different therapies, and I realize that each patient is unique. Assisting patients to recovery has allowed me to hone my communication skills, and I have become adept at teaching while listening and demonstrating compassion. It is hard to verbalize the contentment I feel when I overhear my patients state, "I want that aide again on my next visit."

My role as a physical therapy aide has provided an insider's look into the roles of physician assistants, nurses, doctors, chiropractors, and physical therapists, as well as to the team approach to patient care. After observing different allied health professions closely, I've made an educated decision to pursue the profession of physician assistant. The PA model is the one that best fits my medical interests and career goals. I have witnessed the medical knowledge and expertise required to excel in this field, as well as the listening skills, compassion, and understanding that seem intrinsic in those who are most successful at it.

During high school, I volunteered at a nonprofit home serving low-income persons suffering from HIV/AIDS. Witnessing the mental anguish and physical trauma that these individuals endure was heart wrenching. However, their resilience was remarkable. This experience piqued my interest in the medical field and solidified my desire to help others.

During my junior year, I founded a volunteer chapter called Angel Planes. As president of the organization, I helped organize many successful activities to promote our cause. Our efforts resulted in more than $3,500 in donations to transport children with medical needs and their families to treatment centers.

An effective PA can successfully collaborate with supervising physicians while maintaining their independence and good rapport with patients. I believe they have one of the most unique and rewarding jobs in today's society. Given the opportunity, I am confident I will be an asset to the profession.

The following sections present several annotated essay examples and a selection of paragraphs from essays. The examples may further help you in constructing your own narrative.

Annotated Essay 1

Charles Boelter

The first time I can recall meeting a physician assistant was in the emergency room of Martin Army Community Hospital, at Fort Benning, Georgia. I was a private, going through basic infantry training, and happened to be clumsy enough to fall from the top of the forty-foot rope climb on the obstacle course. I knew he was an officer, but he obviously was neither a doctor nor a nurse. He pulled a large piece of wood from under my thumbnail and sent me for some x-rays. He determined that I was not mortally wounded and released me to my unit.

▲ **Opening paragraph uses a scenario with immediacy to gain the attention of the reader**

I managed to survive basic training, and eventually I wound up as a paratrooper in the 82nd Airborne Division. Throughout the course of my enlistment, I was able to spend a considerable amount of time with our battalion PA.

I learned what he did and what options his profession provided him. When the time came for me to leave active duty, I was beginning to think about the physician assistant profession as a career path.

▲ Outlines interest in the PA profession

I have wanted a career in medicine for as long as I can remember. I am sure this is because of my father and the stories I have heard about him. He learned the intricacies of medicine in school, but he was born with the innate ability to care for and about people.

▲ Identifies a more deeply felt motivation

We lived in a small town, amid a million acres of corn, in rural Illinois. My father practiced from a small office that was actually our converted garage. From the office he took care of the people in our town, on the surrounding farms, and those in the nearby communities. Less than a month after my brother was born, our father left on a house call from which he never returned. He died that night, leaving his sons a legacy of caring and competency that I hear about to this day. My brother never felt the calling of the medical profession as strongly as I have, so he offered encouragement and support to help me achieve my goals. His encouragement stopped when he was killed shortly after I left the military. His death left me as the only one to follow in my father's footsteps.

▲ Strong personal and emotional experiences are stated with restraint

My life has prepared me for a career as a physician assistant in many ways. I believe that, like my father, I have an innate ability to care about people and what happens to them. I want to help make positive changes in their lives much as my father did. Being a leader taught me to be responsible for myself, and for my subordinates. I learned not only how to make decisions but also to recognize the consequences those decisions might have. My work as a medical assistant has given me a better understanding of how the medical team works together to satisfy patient needs. It has exposed me to clinical decision making and the complexities of modern medicine. I have seen firsthand the role physician assistants fulfill in the medical community, and how they fit into the team approach to care, by shadowing them in various settings. I believe I have been given the character and the ability to become a competent physician assistant.

▲ Evidence of self-reflection and understanding of his own skills and abilities

My strongest desire in life is to experience the joys and rigors of a profession in medicine much as my father did. I have the ability and desire to help people, but I need the tools to do this. Becoming a physician assistant will give me the tools I need to take the next step in my career. This is the path I am on, and it is where I can offer the most for those who need help.

▲ **Recaps reasons for wanting to become a PA in a succinct conclusion**

Annotated Essay 2

Yvonne Gonzalez

My interest in becoming a physician associate (PA) is rooted in the desire to provide quality health care to the underprivileged—whose health care needs I have perceived to be acute in the course of my volunteer work. As a social justice coordinator for my parish, I organized volunteer efforts at a number of facilities: pediatric clinics and orphanages in Baja, California, the L.A. Mission and the Catholic Worker (a soup kitchen and free clinic in L.A.). I also represented the parish in a 10-day, 250-mile walkathon from Santa Barbara to Tijuana to raise money for a child welfare agency. I have never felt so much satisfaction in my career achievements as compared to the gratification I derive from working with the underprivileged. Their acute health care needs prompted my desire to become involved in a professional capacity. I felt frustrated, however, because I did not want to become a physician and just could not see myself in any of the allied health careers. It was not until I learned of the physician associate profession that I realized I could fulfill my dream of working in public health at a significant level of medical intervention without having to train for 8 or more years.

▲ **Clear opening sentence paves the way for further supporting evidence**

▲ **Strong history of volunteer work and understanding of social justice issues**

I first learned of physician associates when my father had a double bypass in 1994 and his postoperative care was managed by his cardiologist's staff PA, Helen. When she explained her role to me, I was impressed with the scope of her responsibilities and sensed that this might be the opportunity I had been seeking. Not long after I met Helen, I began shadowing Ted Braunstein, a PA in the emergency department of Mount Sinai Medical Center. I was impressed by his clinical knowledge, compassion, and aptitude for patient education. I was also surprised to see the degree of autonomy given Ted by the attending physicians. We worked out a pact: Ted would answer all of my questions, and I would help him obtain histories and physicals on Spanish-speaking patients. I soon found myself assisting the patient representatives when they were short handed. It wasn't long before I was gloving up to help steady patients as Ted performed suturing of lumbar punctures. Next, the technicians taught me how to draw blood, insert Foley catheters, and take vital measurements. Even after more than 1,500 hours, I am still amazed at the fascinating array of patients and clinical challenges every shift offers.

▲Focuses on initial interest in the profession and builds on how it developed into a life-long goal

▲Uses her own background and language skills to improve patient access to care; specifically lists acquired skills

If given the opportunity, I plan to use my PA training to work in public health. Ideally, I would like to divide my time between an urban tertiary care facility and a rural clinic. Working in such diverse settings will, I feel, provide me with a strong clinical foundation and the opportunity for continuing education that will benefit both patient populations. Serving those in serious need will fulfill a lifelong goal and doing so in a PA capacity will allow me to use the analytical, communication, and time management skills I have acquired in my career thus far. My decision to become a PA is based on a working knowledge of the role of the PA, and I am committed to making the necessary sacrifices to achieve this goal.

▲Presents clear vision of where she wants to be in the future

▲Uses a new slant on her skills to consolidate the essay

Annotated Essay 3

Norman deDios

I have always been fascinated by the mysteries of nature. While my boyhood friends admired Batman, I idolized Jacques Cousteau. To me, he represented man's unrelenting desire to explore the unknown, while demonstrating a deep respect for the natural order of living things. As a child, I consumed countless books on science and spent hours watching documentaries trying to understand the hows and whys of life. I even went so far as to set up my own pet shop in our basement, which eventually contained 100 tropical fish, ranging from a feisty, red-eyed South American manganese to a 2-foot-long silver arrowana. It is this innate curiosity that has evolved into and become the foundation of my desire to study medicine.

▲Strong, unusual beginning paragraph linked to the desire to study medicine

My interest in the natural world took a personal and painful turn when I was awakened to the reality of human beings suffering during my sophomore year at Providence College. At that time, my father suffered a major heart attack, for which he required quadruple bypass surgery and a 4-week stay in hospital. It was frightening to see the man who always seemed invincible to me lying in a hospital attached to so many machines. My father's illness forced me to redefine my role in the family and I suddenly found myself at its head. During that time, I traveled regularly from Providence to New Haven to look after my father and provide support to my mother and siblings. Unfortunately, this sudden shift of responsibility and unfamiliar stress was reflected in my poor grades. The fragility of life and the importance of family became clear to me, and I realized that this difficult period would serve as a transition point toward a new level of maturity, a maturity that strengthened my ability to persevere and heightened my feelings of compassion and concern for others.

▲ A personal experience becomes a turning point

My work experience in health care began with a summer job as a laboratory assistant in the blood chemistry laboratory of the Hospital of Saint Raphael. My responsibilities included keeping records of blood specimens as well as interacting directly with physicians and other members of the hospital staff. The following summer, I was employed as an operating room aide in the ambulatory surgery unit of Yale–New Haven Hospital, where contact with patients on a personal level was a new and rewarding experience. My job gave me the opportunity to interact with patients before their surgery and upon their discharge. It was extremely gratifying to know that the support I offered these patients was not only reassuring but also greatly appreciated. I have always felt a tremendous amount of self-reward knowing that I made a difference in a person's life, simply by showing them I cared. It was this personal time with patients that proved the most satisfying aspect of my job at Yale–New Haven and further motivated me to pursue a career in the health sciences.

▲ Presents another key turning point

After graduating from college, I accepted a position as a research assistant at Yale University School of Medicine, Department of OB-GYN. Working closely with Drs. Aydin Arici and Ibrahim Sozen on their leiomyoma research, I aided in the completion of their study on the effects of growth factor B1 on myometrial tumors. Our work will be published in the near future. After completing my work with Drs. Arici and Sozen, I was given the opportunity to work with David Keefe, also of Yale's OB-GYN department. I thoroughly enjoyed my time with Dr. Keefe due to his confidence in me to work unsupervised and because of the relationship we formed as I occasionally accompanied him throughout his busy day seeing patients. It was with Dr. Keefe that I gained an understanding and appreciation for the intimacy and trust patients have in their health care provider.

▲ Clearly states work outcomes and learning from others

After leaving Yale, I continued to work in the field of research as a laboratory assistant in the Department of Molecular Genetics at New York Medical College. This laboratory was involved in the identification of the gene that caused ataxia telangiectasia, a neuromolecular disease that strikes young children. My responsibilities included cataloging daily blood specimens and isolating DNA for gene identification. Although my role was a small one, it was gratifying to know that my work may aid others in eventually finding a cure for this disease.

While I enjoyed my research, I missed the personal contact I had with patients. This led me to spend this past summer shadowing physician assistants in the cardiothoracic unit at the Hospital of Saint Raphael, which rekindled my interest in clinical medicine. This experience has clarified my image of a physician assistant's role in health care, as well as given me a better understanding of where I hope to be in this field. My interest in patient care has been further enhanced by my current volunteer work with Yale–New Haven Hospital's elder-life program. This position allows me to work one-on-one with geriatric patients and has given me hands-on experience in the health care field. I also feel that volunteer work continues to help me develop techniques for communicating and interacting with patients that I will use in my career as a physician assistant.

▲ Reminds readers of a key factor for wishing to become a PA

Another area in which I have been able to refine my interpersonal skills has been through my involvement in music. At 10 years of age, my friends and I formed a band in which we all continue to perform. As the keyboard player, a vocalist, and a guitarist, I realize that the ability to share and relate ideas is essential to being a successful and unified group. Through music, I have learned the value of patience, cooperation, and understanding, and strive to use these qualities in everyday life.

▲ Provides a good example of transferable skills

I believe that the adversities I have faced have helped me to mature, and I regard them as growing stages in my life. These events have affected me because I genuinely do care about others, and they have shown me how committed and determined I am. I sincerely believe that I possess the qualities to become a responsible, compassionate, and caring physician assistant. Therefore, I refuse to let those obstacles discourage me and to this day I am continuing my education and involvement in health care. I look forward to using my newly found reservoir of strength toward a lifelong career in medicine. My experiences in health care, and my interactions with physician assistants have only strengthened my resolve. I know that as time passes, I can use my experiences, both positive and negative, to become a truly competent physician assistant.

▲ **Clearly reiterates but with a slightly different focus**

ESSAY EXTRACTS

Opening Paragraphs

Imagine waking every day of the year at 4 o'clock in the morning to care for 100 head of dairy cattle. This is what my wife, Carla, and I have done for the past 17 years.
Bradford Phillips

During the past years, I have worked with or shadowed four exceptional physician assistants who have given me valuable insight to the PA profession. As I worked with these health care providers, I analyzed their skills and qualities and inventoried their commonalities. Besides maintaining a high level of technical proficiency, each of them is a superior team leader, outstanding communicator, and creative problem solver. My formal education in psychology and my personal experiences have provided me with an opportunity to develop those three vital qualities.
Amy Fritsch

The inextricable relationship between health and mental health has intrigued me for over 14 years. As a teenager, I watched programs on public television about the etiology of psychotic disorders. After graduating from high school, I decided to follow my natural interests into the world of health care, earning degrees in mental health, psychology, and social work. With each educational milestone, I have gained knowledge and experience that has enhanced my understanding of how to help others in need.
Barbara Ann Slusher

Examples of a Learning Experience that Shaped Individuals' Aspirations

A few years ago, I had occasion to reassess where I was in life and where I had expected to be at that point. I found that the two did not match, and in fact bore little resemblance to each other. It was time to make up my own mind about where and how I spend the rest of my life. The task then became one of determining what track I wanted my life to be on and how I was going to get there. One of the steps in my search led me to volunteer on the neurology/neurosurgery nursing unit at the George Washington University Medical Center—the first volunteer they had ever had. I quickly realized I not only felt very comfortable in the medical environment but also had found a piece of what was missing in my life. Volunteering was good, and quite rewarding, but not nearly enough. I needed to be working in a medical field full-time and be in a position to provide patient care.

Jean Caldwell

The most poignant experience of my career that truly sparked my interest in medicine was my experience as a counselor in a methadone maintenance program. Our treatment team noticed marked improvements in the physical and mental health of our clients after only a short period of methadone treatment. It seemed that heroin addiction was a disease easily treated with methadone. What was confusing, however, was the high rate of relapse for clients who had successfully detoxified from the methadone after years of stable treatment.

Why did clients with such a positive prognosis and years of treatment relapse? We found that many factors influenced a client's ability to remain abstinent from drugs: lifestyle, HIV status, family history, socioeconomic status, et cetera. The relation between these factors was very complex. We could not treat just the physical aspect of the addiction and hope to be successful. For me, this learning experience underlined the fact that disease is not one dimensional. The best treatment approach is one that encompasses the physical, mental, and socioemotional aspects of the individual in their environment.

Barbara Ann Slusher

Although I had various responsibilities at the clinic, what stands out most in my mind was the time I spent listening, counseling, and teaching patients, and the tremendous satisfaction that came from this interaction. One woman I remember came in to see the internist. After a thorough exam and some laboratory tests, the doctor told her that she had diabetes and was going to have to begin insulin therapy. I translated since she spoke only Spanish and could not understand what the doctor was saying. She only asked a few questions and seemed very hesitant and frightened about her future. We reassured her that she was in good hands and we would all be there to support her with the steps she needed to take. A few days later she returned to learn about diabetes management and insulin injections, and again I translated for her. For both the nurse and me it was challenging because she was apprehensive and doubtful that she was going to be able to manage everything by herself. We reassured her that although it was going to be difficult in the beginning, she could do it. We sat with her as she practiced the various tasks, from testing her blood sugar level and giving herself an injection to documenting everything in her journal. After about an hour she was ready to go home, feeling more comfortable with her daily routine. As she left, she took my hand and thanked me for my patience and support, telling me what a good person I was. It seemed strange that she would thank me for this, but her gratitude showed me how important it is to take time to listen, counsel, and support patients.

Katherine Coleman

Example of a Strong Conclusion

These volunteer experiences have crystallized the challenges, rewards, and frustrations of being a health care provider, as well as the shortcomings of health care in the United States. These diverse environments have augmented my studies in public health, and have provided me with concrete examples of how individuals can benefit from caring, sensitive providers, and how communities suffer when adequate health care services are not available or affordable. As a physician assistant I will be poised to deliver health care services to under-served urban populations, and I will demonstrate compassion and sensitivity. Furthermore, the intensive, rigorous PA program at . . . will enable me to execute this career change effectively and efficiently.

Lynn R. Fryer

Work History Sheet

Employer name: _____

Address: _____

Phone: _____

Full time: _____ Part time: _____

Dates of employment: From: _____ To:_____

Job title: _____

Job description: (3 sentences or less) _____

_____

_____

Skills ultilized: _____

Awards/citations: _____

Other information: _____

Medical Experience Sheet

Employer name: _____

Address: _____

Phone: _____

No. of months worked: Full time: _____ Part time: _____

Dates of employment: From: _____ To:_____

Job title: _____

Job description: (3 sentences or less) _____

_____

Skills ultilized (e.g. phlebotomy, vital signs, physical exams):

_____

Awards/citations: _____

Describe your most memorable patient (3 sentences or less):

_____

_____

Other information: _____

_____

High School Information Sheet

High school attended: _____

Address: _____

Dates attended: From: _____ To: _____

GPA: _____

Team sports: _____

Clubs: _____

Awards/honors: _____

Volunteer work: _____

Other: _____

College Information Sheet

College/university attended: _____

Address: _____

Dates attended: From: _____ To: _____

Major: _____

Highest degree obtained: _____

GPA: _____

Team sports: _____

Clubs: _____

Awards/honors: _____

Volunteer work: _____

Did you work?: yes_____ no_____

List one person whom you can contact for a good reference:

_____

Scholarships: _____

Other: _____

Volunteer Work

Volunteer description: _____

Why this position?: _____

Address: _____

Point of contact: _____

How long?: _____

Awards/letters of appreciation: _____

_____

Most memorable patient: _____

_____

List one person who will write a good reference for you: _____

_____

Military Service

Branch of service: _____

Dates of service: _____

Type of discharge: _____

Where stationed?: _____

Job title (M.O.S.): _____

Supervisor: _____

Awards/ribbons/medals: _____

_____

Special schools/training: _____

_____

Did you attend college in the military?: _____

What did you learn from the experience?: _____

_____

Foreign Language

Do you speak a foreign language?: _____

What language? _____

How did you learn the language?: _____

_____

Travel

Where to?: _____

When?: _____

What did you learn from the experience? _____

_____

_____

Special Awards/Citations

Award type: _____

Why received?: _____

When received?: _____

Given by: _____

What did you do to get it? _____

_____

CHAPTER 7

The Interview (Part One)

The next three chapters focus on various aspects of the interview process. In this chapter, I focus on some of the necessary skills you must have or acquire to be a strong applicant. I also provide you with some insight into the interview process from the perspective of an applicant who failed on her first try but was accepted the next year. In Chapter 8, I provide an overview of the interview process and teach you how to prepare for it. I'll explain the different types of interviews (group, individual, and student) and introduce you to the scoring process. In Chapter 9, I provide you with actual interview questions and answers so you can maximize your preparation for the big day.

INTRODUCTION

Every PA school receives hundreds of applications each year. Once your application is received, the registrar will check it for completeness and forward it on for review by the admissions committee. Two committee members will review your application, give you a numerical score, and make a decision as to your interview status. Most programs invite approximately 100 applicants to interview. There is only one program that I am aware of that does not interview; Cuyahoga Community College in Ohio uses an extensive questionnaire to screen and evaluate candidates for acceptance.

It is important to mention that an applicant should not be too aggressive in seeking an interview. **Never call a PA program to request or**

demand an interview. The decision to interview a candidate rests solely with the admissions committee. The committee does not look favorably on students who call to request or demand an interview. In fact, each time you contact the program and speak with an administrator, a note is usually placed in your file as to the reason for the call. You certainly do not want any unfavorable information placed in your file that will compromise your chances for acceptance. You may call the program to inquire whether you will be invited for an interview but only after the application deadline has passed by several weeks.

HOW IMPORTANT IS THE INTERVIEW?

At this point in the application process, you should realize that the interview is all that counts. Everything else—your education, work experience, essay, test scores—simply support this crucial meeting. Remember that statistics are cold and cerebral. Just because you have a 4.0 grade point average and you scored 1,400 on your SATs does not mean that you will automatically be accepted into PA school.

The admissions committee wants to learn more about you as a person. Are you likable? Are you compassionate? Do you fully understand the role of the PA? Are you mature? Can you handle stress? Can the interviewer visualize you as a colleague? Are you overconfident? Are you trustworthy? Are you energetic? Would the interviewer want you taking care of him or her as a patient? Are you an effective communicator? The interview is your chance to sell yourself to the committee. Your grades, SAT scores, and essay were already good enough to get you this far. It is now time to concentrate on making an emotional connection with all of the committee members.

HIGH-IMPACT COMMUNICATION

To win a position in next year's class, you need to develop certain skills and behaviors that will enhance your position. The first of these behaviors is charisma, or extraordinary personal power or charm. To some, charisma comes naturally, but more often than not, it must be learned. Charisma is the result of a series of behaviors through which someone has a powerful and positive impact on others. This is exactly what you want to accomplish at the interview; use charisma to build the bridge to credibility and trust.

I interviewed many applicants who simply could not make a connection at the interview. Those applicants could not move beyond facts, figures, and jargon to make a connection. In contrast, the applicants who scored the highest at the interview knew how to communicate effectively and persuasively, and above all, they were absolutely believable. They understood how to project openness, enthusiasm, and energy. **The ability to communicate effectively is the single most important skill you need to succeed as a PA.**

Communication is a contact sport. As mentioned already, looking good on paper will get you only so far. If you are unable to make an emotional connection with your audience, you're likely to be rejected. I witnessed this phenomenon over and over again when I interviewed applicants. Although some candidates were only average on paper, they made such an emotional impact at the interview that I scored them higher than I had anticipated on the basis of their application alone.

CREATING EMOTIONAL IMPACT

You must learn to sell yourself to create emotional impact. While preparing for one of my seminars, I received an e-mail from a person on the staff of a PA program in the southern United States. He wanted to "join the team" and help me out with my upcoming seminar in his location. I wrote back thanking him for his interest but told him that I was not looking to hire anyone at that point. A week later, I received a telephone call from another PA wanting to come aboard and help me out with my seminars. That person, Chris, told me that he had seven years' experience on one of the local PA programs' admissions committees. He sold me on the idea that he would truly be an asset to my seminar program. He understood the power of the living résumé versus sending an e-mail. Chris understood that he was selling himself, and I offered him a position.

What are you selling? Have you thought about it? Some people get uncomfortable when I mention the word *selling*. They fail to realize that we all sell ourselves every day. We sell our ideas to our employers. We sell our crucial decisions to our spouses and loved ones. You will have to sell yourself to the admissions committee and give them a reason to invite you into the next class of PA school students.

The Secret

If I can get you to buy into the fact that we are all selling something, then you must also understand this crucial point: **The admissions committee**

selects candidates on the basis of emotion and justifies its decision with facts. If you can grasp this secret, you will realize why I emphasize that you cannot rely on your paper application to be accepted; you must make an emotional connection with the committee.

After you walk out of the interview room, the committee doesn't sit down with a legal pad and draw a line down the center separating your strengths and weaknesses. Your score, and the ultimate decision of whether to accept you into the program, is mainly influenced by emotional factors rather than rational factors alone. If committee members liked you at an emotional level, they will justify giving you a higher score by commenting favorably on your grade point average, SAT scores, medical experience, or whatever will work to support this emotionally based decision. If the committee doesn't like you at an emotional level, you can have a 4.0 grade point average and 1,400 SAT scores and still not win their support.

Three Key Points to Remember

Creating emotional impact is crucial to your success as a PA school applicant. Personal impact is power—power to achieve whatever you want in your personal life and career. Consider these three key points prior to your interview:

1. The spoken word is almost the exact opposite of the written word
The written word is a one-dimensional medium for communicating facts and transferring information. The spoken word, however, is multidimensional and includes a kaleidoscope of nonverbal cues such as posture, eye contact, energy, volume, intonation, and much more. If you want to make an emotional impact and motivate and persuade the admissions committee, you must master the spoken word and learn to make such nonverbal cues work for you rather than against you.

2. What you say must be believed for it to have an impact
If the committee senses that you are less than forthright with even one interview question, you will build a wall of distrust that you probably will not be able to overcome. For your message to be believed, you must be believed.

I once interviewed a woman who was an accomplished actress. She presented the committee with a very fancy and off-beat resume. Located on the bottom right-hand corner of the resume, below all of her Off-Broadway credits, she wrote, "Special Talents: I can tie a cherry stem into a knot with my tongue." Although this particular talent may be relevant to her role as an actress, it was completely inappropriate for a PA school application, and she had already lost her credibility with me and my fellow interviewers before she stepped foot into the interview room. One of my colleagues who wasn't too pleased with that note on her résumé asked the applicant to comment on her most memorable patient. The applicant started to cry. My colleague asked her, point blank, "How do we know you're not acting now?" The candidate became very silent.

People's gut feeling as to whether they like and believe someone is usually based on emotion, not logic. If your voice cracks, or your hands are fidgety, or you cannot make solid eye contact, you'll probably lose credibility with your audience.

3. Believability is determined at the subconscious level

Perhaps this is the most important point to remember. How do we determine whether we believe someone? Can you build believability out of a mountain of facts and figures? Absolutely not. You cannot even build trust out of a stack of eloquently crafted words. Authoritative credentials, a title, or a letter of recommendation from a big shot may give you a little credibility and get you to the interview, but you still have to be believable to close the sale.

How do you make yourself more believable? First, you must make eye contact. Without good eye contact the committee members may become suspicious of you and wonder what you are hiding. Be sure to smile. Don't become so self-involved and nervous that you forget to relax and smile. **Smiling is infectious and will help you and the committee members relax. Use open gestures.** Don't sit at the table with your arms folded tightly over your chest. Keep your arms and hands open, which will support the fact that you are an open-minded person. Use a firm handshake. There is nothing worse than a wet, limp handshake. Finally, have good posture and project a strong voice.

Interviewers are Bombarded with Visual Stimuli that Register at the Preconscious Level

From the moment we walk into the interview, we begin giving off a series of verbal and nonverbal cues. Do you walk into a room tall, or do you slump? Do you have a firm handshake? Do you refer to your patients as legs and arms, or do you refer to them by name? Do you refer to nurses in a derogatory manner, or do you give them the respect they deserve?

An enormous amount of communication is taking place as thousands of multichannel impressions are carried to the brain. Most impressions register at the preconscious level. As a result of the impressions, the brain forms a continuous stream of emotional judgments and assessments: Do I trust this person? Is she honest, evasive, threatening, friendly? Is he interesting, boring, warm, cold, anxious? Is she confident, insecure, or perhaps hiding something?

The emotional judgment that forms in your preconscious mind about the speaker determines whether you will tune in or tune out to his or her message. If you distrust someone at the emotional level, little of what that person says will get through.

Getting to Trust

How do we use our natural self to reach the emotional center of our listeners? **You've got to be believed to be heard.** When dealing with the admissions committee, trust and believability are synonymous. You can't have one without the other. To communicate effectively with the committee, they must trust you. And to win their trust, you must be believable. Belief occurs at the gut level; it's acceptance on faith, it's emotionally based, and it bypasses the intellect.

During the interview, each committee member sifts through your nuances of behavior. Does your voice quiver, or does it project authority? Do your eyes flicker hesitantly or gaze unflinchingly? Is your posture confident or diffident? These nuances of behavior speak the language of trust.

People learn as babies who they trust and why. One day my son Eddie and I were at the airport on our way to Orlando, Florida, where I was to present a seminar. While sitting in the chairs by our gate, a toddler playfully strolled over to us with a smile on her face from ear to ear. She was cooing and drooling and having a grand old time. Eddie and I played peekaboo with her, causing her to shriek with laughter and excitement. Then she suddenly strolled over to a man sitting next to us and smiled playfully at him. Without saying a word, he gave her a look that said, "I'm not interested in you little girl. Go away!" The little girl's face went from a huge smile to a little pout. She ran from the man and knew that he represented trouble; he wasn't safe.

You cannot communicate with a baby using words. Instead, infants relate to facial expressions, energy, and sound. A baby responds with the same set of verbal cues. The smile is the language of our emotional centers. Even a baby knows that a person who doesn't smile lacks warmth and safety. We learn early in life that the people we should trust are those who (genuinely) smile. To communicate effectively, we must relearn the language of trust.

Did you ever meet someone and instantly like or dislike that person but not know why? When you meet someone for the first time, the emotional center in your brain receives thousands of nonverbal cues that are registered at the preconscious level. Your intuition comes from this; you form an almost-immediate impression of that person. You form an impression that is detailed and often richly colored with emotion.

Most candidates approach the interview as though their essay, grades, and SAT scores are what count most. They fail to realize that when they leave that interview, the individual committee members don't comment on logic and reason. Rather, they typically say, "I like her," or "I don't believe him," or "There's something about her that I really like."

Some people can naturally do this without understanding how it works. The candidate who knows how to speak the language of the brain's emotional center—the language of trust—is the candidate most likely to be believed and accepted. That language communicates very rapidly and effectively.

The Likability Factor

In 1984, President Reagan ran for reelection against Walter Mondale. A Gallup Poll examined three areas with respect to each candidate: (1) issues, (2) party affiliation, and (3) likability. On the issues, the candidates were considered dead even. The Democrat clearly had the edge when it came to party affiliation. With respect to likability, however, Reagan had the edge and won the election. It was the personality factor that dominated.

As applicants, we pride ourselves on having a great grade point average, test scores, and years of hands-on medical experience. But when it's time to interview, it's your likability that determines whether you receive a letter of acceptance or a letter of rejection. As soon as you walk into that interview room, it's the visual connection that sets the beginning of trust and believability.

The Eye Factor

The eye is the only sensory organ that contains brain cells. Memory experts invariably link the objects they remember to a visual image. Research shows that it's the visual image that makes the greatest impact in communication.

Researchers generally agree that the spoken word is made up of three components: the verbal, the vocal, and the visual. The verbal message, or the actual words that we use, are what most people concentrate on, but this is actually the most insignificant part of the spoken message. The vocal component is made up of the intonation, projection, and resonance of your spoken message. **It is the visual message, however, the emotion and expression of your body and face as you speak, that carries the most weight.**

This professor also found that the degree of consistency or inconsistency among those three elements determines the believability of your message. The more the three factors harmonize, the more believable you are as a candidate. If your verbal message is not in harmony with your body language, you send a mixed signal to the emotional center of the other person's brain. Your message may or may not get through to the decision-making, rational portion of your brain. The three components of the spoken message are quantified as follows:

- Verbal = 7%
- Voice = 38%
- Visual = 55%

In other words, what you see is what you get. If you come into the interview room yawning or dressed inappropriately, nothing you do or say will help you. The interviewer is likely to shut you out immediately and not hear a word you have to say.

HOW DO YOU ENHANCE YOUR MESSAGE?

Eye Contact

The first way to enhance your communication is with eye contact. This is the number-one skill you should develop before you interview. Three rules and exercises for maintaining eye contact follow

Rules
1. Use involvement rather than intimacy or intimidation.
2. Count to five (involvement), then look away.
3. Don't dart your eyes; this represents a lack of confidence.

Exercises
1. **Use video feedback.** Tape yourself speaking with someone and watch for your use of, or violation of, the three rules.

2. **Practice one-on-one.** Have a conversation with someone you trust and ask that person for direct feedback with respect to the rules.

3. **Practice with a paper audience.** Draw smiley faces on sticky notes and then place them on a chair and practice making eye contact, counting to five, and looking away.

Posture and Movement

The next way to enhance your message is with posture and movement. **A good posture commands attention, and movement shows confidence.** Walk into the room standing tall. Don't slump. When you speak to your interviewer, don't be afraid to add movement to your message. You don't have to wave your hands all over the room, but use open gestures to come across as a friendly, open-minded person. Four rules for posture are:

Rules

1. Stand tall.
2. Watch your lower body; don't lean back on one hip or rock back and forth.
3. Get in the ready position; lean slightly forward if you're sitting or on the balls of your feet if you're standing.
4. Use movement to show that you're excited, enthusiastic, and confident.

Exercises

1. **Walk away from the wall.** Stand with your back against a wall, heels pressed against the wall along with your head, neck, and shoulders. Try to push the small of your back into the wall. Now simply walk away from the wall and feel how upright and correct your posture becomes. Try to shake off this posture; you can't. Practice this exercise daily so that when you walk into the interview room, you'll command attention.

2. **Use the ready position.** Remember, if you're standing, sit up slightly on the balls of your feet. If you are sitting, lean slightly forward toward the interviewer.

Dress and Appearance

The third way to enhance your message is with dress and appearance. **You get only two seconds to make your initial impression on your interviewers.** If you blow it, it may take more than 30 minutes to recover, and most interviews last for only 20 minutes. So, it is critical to make a good first impression.

When you dress up for an interview, only 10% of your skin should show. Be sure that your face is well shaven or your makeup is not too overbearing. Comb or style your hair, avoid wearing extravagant jewelry, clean and trim your nails, and use cologne or perfume sparingly.

Rules

1. Be appropriate—when in Rome . . .
2. Be conservative; when in doubt, dress up.
3. Men, always button your jacket.
4. Don't do overkill on perfume or cologne.
5. Always bring a small mirror and check your face before interviewing.

Exercises

1. **Get feedback.** Ask friends and relatives how well you present yourself. Be open to constructive criticism.
2. **Be observant; read fashion magazines.** Find a style with which you are comfortable. Don't go over the edge, however.

Gestures and Smile

The final way to enhance your message is with gestures and your smile. **Do you speak with conviction, enthusiasm, and passion?** Are you friendly or stuffy? Do you speak with open gestures and a warm smile, or are you a fig-leaf flasher, always covering and uncovering your groin with your hands. Remember, openness equals likability. Here are 3 rules for gestures and smiling:

Rules

1. Be aware of nervous gestures and stop them.
2. Lift the apples of your cheeks—smile. Make believe that you have apples on your cheekbones and try to lift them up to your forehead.
3. Feel your smile, but beware: Phony smiles don't work.

Exercises

1. **Imitate someone whom you feel is an effective communicator and play the part with gusto.** Get used to using open gestures and expressions.
2. **Be natural.** Incorporate some of these gestures into your daily communication.

THE ENERGY FACTOR

Energy is the fuel that drives the car of success. You don't want to run out of gas when you're halfway up the hill. Think back to the last morning that you awoke feeling completely refreshed, like you could conquer the world. Wasn't that a powerful space to be in? That place is exactly where you need to be on the day of the interview—in the zone. This section focuses on ways to unlock your inner energy and present yourself in the best light to the admissions committee.

Voice and Vocal Variety

Use intonation and inflection in your voice. **Speaking in a monotone can be deadly and can put your listeners to sleep.** Observe and practice the following rules and exercises to add energy to your voice.

Rules

1. Make your voice naturally authoritative; speak from the diaphragm.
2. Put your voice on a roller coaster; practice reading from magazines using intonation and inflection.
3. Be aware of your telephone voice; it represents 84% of the emotional impact when people can't see you.
4. Smile when talking on the telephone; people can feel your smile right through the phone.
5. Put your real feelings into your voice.

Exercises

1. **Breathe from the diaphragm.** Take in a deep breath from your nose and let it out slowly, stopping to feel the pressure on your diaphragm. This is where a strong voice originates.

2. **Project your voice.** Try speaking in a normal voice first, and then project your voice so it reaches the back of the room. Try to find the right depth in your voice without straining your vocal chords.

3. **Practice varying your pitch and pace.** Read from magazines.

Words and Nonwords

Energize with words and avoid using nonwords that are meaningless and take away from your message.

Rules

1. Build your vocabulary, especially with synonyms (see Appendix D).
2. Paint word pictures. Create motion and emotion with metaphors.
3. Beware of jargon, especially medical jargon. Say "operating room" instead of "OR"
4. Avoid meaningless nonwords like *ah* and *um*, or words used to stall like *so*, *well*, and *you know*. Replace those words with a silent pause. A properly timed pause adds drama, energy, and power to your message. Try listening to the voice of the famous commentator Paul Harvey. He is the master of the pause and has made a career out of using the technique.

Listener Involvement

Humans communicate, and books dispense information. Try using the following techniques to add an extra punch to your communication.

Rules

1. Use a strong opening. Make it visual and energetic by including pauses, action and motion, and joy and laughter.
2. Maintain eye communication. When you enter the room for a group interview, survey your listeners for 3 to 5 seconds, gauge, and adjust.
3. Lean toward your listeners.
4. Create interest by maintaining eye contact and having high energy.

Use Humor Effectively

"I will not make age an issue in this campaign. I will not exploit my opponent's youth and inexperience." Those words changed an entire campaign in Ronald Reagan's favor, after he spoke them at a national debate with Walter Mondale. In reference to an age question he anticipated, Reagan was prepared with that witty response, which turned out to be the most remembered sentences uttered at the debate.

I do not recommend that you tell jokes at your interview, and remember that fun is better than funny. The goal is not comedy but connection. Find the form of humor that works for you, and be natural.

KARIN'S EXPERIENCE

Before next chapter's overview of the actual interview process, let's take a look at what one of my friends and colleagues has to say about her interview experience at Yale University. Karin Augur did not get accepted the first year she applied; however, after making some adjustments, she reapplied the next year and was accepted. Her experience offers a great deal of insight into the interview process.

> Applying to PA school or any other graduate school can be a very stressful process. Knowing yourself and the profession you are striving to enter are two of the most important factors in the application process. This is particularly evident during the interview. To be absolutely sure that a career as a physician assistant is what you truly desire, you must have an in-depth and intimate knowledge of what a physician assistant does. Conveying that knowledge and your passion for the profession to the interviewer will translate to a successful interview.
>
> When applying to PA school, an impressive application is always important. Once you are granted an interview, demonstrating your attributes in person is even more important. The interviewers are looking for someone with strong character, good communication skills, and focused goals. Even with mediocre qualifications on paper, an impressive interview can significantly increase your chances of being accepted.
>
> My first attempt at PA school proved to be a painful eye-opener. After graduating from one of the top five schools in the country, having earned a BA in biology, I was convinced that pursuing a Ph.D. for a career in research was my calling in life. After several months working in a cell biology laboratory, I realized this was not my life dream. I soon began volunteering at a university emergency department, where I first encountered a physician assistant. Immediately, I knew that career path was one that I would enjoy, and I began preparing to enter PA school. I filled out all of the applications and mentally began to prepare for the interviews. During that year of preparation, I also became engaged to my current husband and found myself preparing for a

wedding. As you can imagine, the year was quite hectic and emotionally over-whelming. One by one I heard from each of the schools, and to my utter sur-prise, I was rejected by all of them. I could not believe it. What had happened? After the initial shock subsided, I soon realized why I was denied acceptance.

Despite being physically present at the various interviews, I was not present in spirit. Besides being distracted by my wedding plans, I had not fully let go of the idea of a career in research. The following year, I not only had to deal with a bruised ego but I was also forced to take a long, hard look at myself. I continued doing research and volunteering in the emergency department. I decided to start shadowing a PA and realized I had a lot more to learn about the profession. I quickly embraced the idea that, yes, I wanted to be a PA. I focused my energy on improving myself as an applicant. As a result, I was accepted to my school of choice. I completed the program in two years, finishing second in my class.

Whatever your goals are in life, you must embrace them fully. This is what I learned during my application and interview process. This is exactly what went wrong the first year I applied. Understanding your individual strengths and weaknesses and improving upon them are an excellent way to make you a stronger applicant. Learning as much as you can about physician assistants and how you as an individual will satisfy your dreams is as important to your inter-view as it is to your lifelong happiness.

[CHAPTER 8]

The Interview
(Part Two)

This chapter covers an overview of the interview process and gives you a feel for what to expect. In addition, I provide you with 21 tips to help you excel in your interview.

OVERVIEW OF THE INTERVIEW PROCESS

Not all interviews are conducted in the same fashion. The following descriptions represent only a sample of what you may face on interview day.

When you get up on the morning of your interview, and before you even get out of bed, ask yourself this question: What is the worst thing that could possibly happen today? Once you think about the answer to this question and accept that you will still have your life, health, and family at the end of the day, you will feel more relaxed and able to perform to your potential.

Once you arrive at the interview location, someone from the PA program staff will greet you. Whoever that person is, be sure to smile, shake hands, and be polite. You are now officially being evaluated, and that process will continue until you leave in the afternoon or evening.

You will be directed to a room in which other interviewees may be seated (unless you're the first to arrive, of course). Again, you should smile, shake hands, and introduce yourself to everyone. Even if someone walks in after you, be the first to extend a handshake and a hello. Remember, you are being evaluated all day, and this is a good way to show off some of your good qualities.

It is a good idea to speak with everyone—ask them about their background, where else they have interviewed, where they are from, and so on. Allow others to speak, too. The key is to not be too shy or obnoxious. Find the balance, and above all, be genuine.

After everyone arrives, you likely will begin a short series of talks with the director of the program, the director of admissions, and the financial aid officer. Listen intently, ask intelligent questions, and stay relaxed. Do not feel that you have to dominate the situation; you'll have time to shine when the actual interviews start.

Next up are the case scenarios. These are a set of three to four written questions that everyone will have about fifteen minutes to answer. They are not meant to stress you out before the interview; they are simply a way to get an idea of your ability to reason and make sound judgments.

Once you've finished the case scenarios, you'll be split up into two groups; half will begin the interview process, and half will attend a class with the first-year students. When you go to the class, remember that you are always being evaluated. Inappropriate comments to students can ruin your day. Pay attention to the lecture; remember the instructor's name; and ask sensible, relevant questions only if you feel it is absolutely necessary to do so. If you'd like, you can ask the students questions before and after the class.

At most programs, the interviews consist of three parts: the student interview, the group interview, and the single interview. There are usually two students, a first year and a second year, in the student interview. The group interview consists of three PAs or MDs, and the single interviewer is usually the senior PA or a psychologist or psychiatrist. **Keep in mind, though, that not all programs follow the same interview patterns or procedures.**

After the morning interviews, you'll have lunch, meet with some of the current students, and then switch roles with the other applicants. If you have already interviewed, do not make any comments about the questions or process.

At the end of the day, you will likely all be offered a tour of the facility. We recommend that you take this tour unless you have a flight or train to catch. If that's the case, let the leader of the interview group know that you have to keep to your schedule, and thank him or her for the opportunity to interview. If you go on the tour, ask intelligent questions; don't fool around; and most important, ask yourself whether it seems like the kind of place where you'd like to go to school.

THE STUDENT INTERVIEW

Although the student interview tends to be the most relaxed interview, let your guard down and you could find yourself reapplying next year. The students take this interview very seriously, and they could make you or break you. They usually do not have access to all of your application, but they score you and comment on your performance. They basically want to know three things about you:

1. Do you know what a PA is and does?
2. Have you worked as hard as they have to get here?
3. Would you make a good classmate?

Keep in mind that students tend to grade tougher than the committee members. Remember in grade school when the teacher allowed the students to grade their own papers? People are usually much tougher on themselves. Students have a great sense of pride in their accomplishments, their school, and the PA profession. Don't blow it by making comments like "You're only students" or "The hard part is over; you guys will be easy." You might as well say good-bye.

A good tip is to ask the students what they like about the program and why they like it. Ask them why you should pick this school, if given the opportunity, over Duke, Yale, or Emory, for example. Let them sell you a little bit.

THE GROUP INTERVIEW

For some, this is the toughest part of the day. I've seen applicants cry, get mad, clam up, shake, rattle, and roll in the group interview. In the group interview, you usually have three or more committee members, usually PAs and MDs, who have just reread your application and have specific and general questions in mind. The committee has six basic things to find out from you:

1. Do you have a good concept of the PA profession?
2. Can you handle the program academically?
3. Will you fit in with the class, and will you be able to contribute to it?
4. Are you a compassionate person?

5. Are you a team player?

6. Can you handle the stress of the program?

It is your job to convince the group that the answer is yes on all accounts. We will cover the questions, and specific answers, in Chapter 9.

The group has no hidden agenda; they're really not trying to trip you up. Some applicants become very defensive when asked certain questions. Remain cool; never raise your voice; and as the commercial says, never let them see you sweat. The committee wants you to do well; some of them may have even originally scored your application to get you there.

The following are some general tips for interviewing:

- Be honest.
- Be genuine.
- If you don't know the answer, admit it.
- Don't beg to be accepted.
- Think! Think! Think!
- Smile.
- Make eye contact.

Once the group interview is over, you'll be asked if you have any questions. See the end of the chapter for a short list of appropriate questions to ask the committee. You do not have to ask questions. In fact, the committee will not care one way or the other if you ask questions or not. The exception is asking too many questions at the interview or asking inappropriate questions. **Before you leave the room, be sure to thank each member of the group by name.**

THE INDIVIDUAL INTERVIEW

The purpose of this interview is threefold:

1. To verify what you have told the other interviewers.

2. To see whether your answers are consistent.

3. To find out more about your personal life.

Be consistent with your answers. If you have done your homework, you'll have no problem. For instance, don't think that you can tell the students and the group interviewers that you never thought of going to medical school, and then confide in the single interviewer that you applied twice but weren't accepted. This is inconsistent and likely to lower your score.

If you draw a psychologist for your single interview, he or she may ask you very personal questions. Don't get flustered. Don't volunteer too much information either. Avoid talking about drugs, sexual preference, the family alcoholic, and topics that may get you into trouble. If they hand you a rope, don't hang yourself with it.

SCORING AND RATING YOUR INTERVIEW

After each interview session, morning and afternoon, the entire committee meets to discuss the candidates, compare notes, and give you a score. You may be rated in six areas; within those, each committee may decide on common indicators that best summarize the qualities of a good PA.

1. Cognitive and Verbal Ability

The committee will want to know whether you have the ability to think through a problem and respond appropriately. Are you a lifelong learner? Can you articulate your ideas in a logical sequence? How perceptive are you about others? Here, both verbal ability and written skills are important indicators. The committee will also want to see evidence of your organizational skills, for instance, time management strategies or your ability to prioritize, and indeed your problem-solving processes. You will need to show, too, that you understand the rigor of the PA program of study.

2. Motivation to Become a PA

Are you strongly motivated or just testing the waters? Why do you want to become a PA? Are you interested in patients or the science of medicine? The committee will want to get a sense of your enthusiasm and commitment to the profession. You will need to demonstrate that you are a practical person who has had experience with patient care.

3. Understanding of the PA Profession

Do you know what PA practice entails? Do you know any PAs? Have you worked with any PAs? In this area, the committee will look to see whether you are realistic in your understanding of the role of a PA and that you have a positive attitude toward nurses and doctors. Once again, the committee will be interested in how patient-oriented you are.

4. Interpersonal Skills and Behavior

Do you work collaboratively? Will patients and colleagues respect you? Or, do you come across as too eager and domineering? Are you courteous and tactful in dealing with others? Are you compassionate? There is a range of key areas within this category, from good grooming and personal presentation to more complex communication skills, that the panel will look at to see that you demonstrate appropriate listening skills, have an understanding of different audiences, are warm and open without being overly friendly, and can be diplomatic when required. Obviously, coming across as too aggressive or fabricating your experience to win points will not score you points with the panel.

5. Ability to Handle Stress

Except for being a bit nervous in the interview, is it clear that you can relax and be at ease? Do you have a sense of humor? Are you articulate? Do you convey your ideas clearly? Do you remain poised and relatively calm in the face of stressful situations? Do you have a measure of self-possession? Are you overanxious or confused in times of stress?

6. Personal Characteristics

Are you thoughtful and innovative? Are you a technician or a decision maker? Are the facts you present in your interview consistent with your written file? Some of the key areas that a panel may look for here are your level of maturity, self-drive, and determination balanced with flexibility and creativity. Your ability to empathize with others is also an important indicator in this area.

Each program has its own rating system. For instance, a 10-point scale may be used, with 10 being the best (accept) and 1 being the worst (reject), or a scale that places applicants in one of the following categories: definite acceptance, probable acceptance, uncertain, probable rejection, definite rejection. After each session of interviews is over, the committee meets to give the final scores. An applicant's name is called, and each committee member will simply call out his or her score. Once the scores are collected on all of the applicants, the discussions begin. Again, each program has its own method of evaluating interviewees.

If an applicant scores all 1s or all 10s, there's nothing to discuss. Most applicants, however, fall somewhere in the middle and require further discussion. For instance, if the students score an applicant 10 and 10, respectively; the group scores the applicant 10, 8, and 10, respectively; and the single interviewer scores the same applicant 4, there's obviously a problem here. What does the single interviewer know that the rest of the committee doesn't?

Upon asking the single interviewer why he or she gave the student a 4, we may find out that everything went well until the applicant mentioned his problems with drugs and alcohol. There is a problem that this interviewer uncovered. At this point, the students and group change their scores and the applicant does not get in.

The process can also work in reverse. Someone may really champion an applicant and convince everyone else to give a better score. There are an extensive number of checks and balances set up to be sure that only the best candidates get accepted.

INTERVIEWING TIPS AND RULES

1. Arrive to the interview on time.
2. Dress appropriately. Men should wear a suit and tie, women should wear a suit, and men and women should have their shoes shined.
3. Bring a compact mirror to quickly look over your face.
4. Smile genuinely.
5. Always offer your (firm) handshake first.
6. Look everyone in the eyes.
7. Speak clearly and loudly enough to be heard.
8. Use proper English.
9. Say "please" and "thank you."
10. Don't sit until asked to do so.
11. Bring a copy of your entire application; review it when you have free time.
12. Prepare a short list of good questions to ask.

13. Bring a picture of yourself.
14. When interviewing, try not to make nervous hand movements.
15. Don't become defensive.
16. Don't ever raise your voice.
17. Don't say too much.
18. Listen to everyone with genuine interest.
19. Be consistent.
20. Answer the question briefly.
21. Don't ramble.

GOOD QUESTIONS TO ASK

After you finish each interview, you will be given the opportunity to ask questions. You do not have to ask any questions, and if you don't, it's not likely to count against you. But if you ask inappropriate questions or too many questions, you're liable to annoy the interviewers. If you choose not to ask any questions, simply say, "No thank you. I've had all of my questions answered already." If you do ask questions, use the following list as a guide:

For Students
- What do you like best about this program?
- Why should I pick this program over any other program?
- What do you like least about this program?

For the Group
- If I'm selected, why should I pick this program over a different school?
- What is this school's first-time pass-fail rate on the national boards?
- What is the highlight of this program?

For the Single Interviewer
- Why is this program so successful?
- What can be improved about this program?
- What is this school's first-time pass-fail rate on the boards?

Do Not Ask

- So, what do you do for excitement?
- How's the partying around here?
- Are there lots of women/men here?

AFTER THE INTERVIEW

After you go home from the interview, write a letter of thanks (not an e-mail) to the director of the program. This will be placed in your file, whether or not you get in. If it's the latter, it may help you next year.

CHAPTER 9

The Interview (Part Three)

In Chapter 8, we focused on the interview process and the particular skills you should exhibit to perform well. In this chapter, we focus on the exact questions that you are likely to be asked, and I provide an insider's slant on what the committee really wants to know.

Too many applicants feel that they can come to the interview and just wing it. This can be a fatal mistake. In a climate of hundreds of applicants for too-few slots, you must practice, practice, practice. If you don't, you may find yourself applying again next year.

I do not recommend that you memorize the exact answers to the questions I give here. This, too, can be a fatal mistake. Rather, I encourage you to incorporate the concepts into your own experiences and formulate answers that are specific to you and your situation.

The questions and answers in this chapter will be set up in this format:

- Question:
- In other words:
- Answer:

The first six areas of questions cover the areas discussed in the previous chapter on scoring and rating your interview. The remainder includes more questions that you could likely be asked. Keep your answers short but concise.

COGNITIVE AND VERBAL ABILITY

Question: How has your academic work prepared you for the PA profession?

In other words: Can you handle the rigor of our didactic phase?

Answer: If you have filled out the worksheets from Chapter 6, you will be well prepared to answer this question. "I have a BS in chemistry with a 3.3 GPA. In addition, I recently completed a microbiology course and anatomy and physiology, and I received an A in each class. Throughout college, I worked at a part-time job and volunteered at the local hospital." This applicant not only demonstrates the ability to handle difficult science coursework; he or she also demonstrates good time management skills and the ability to do more than one thing at a time.

Question: Tell us about the last book you read.

In other words: Tell us something about yourself—your interests.

Answer: You may not want to mention that you read the latest Danielle Steel novel. Play it safe: "I just read a biography of Abraham Lincoln. He surmounted incredible odds to become president. It was a very inspiring story."

Question: What is the most important issue facing the health care system in the United States?

In other words: Can you articulate an intelligent response to an area that affects all of us as citizens and as health care workers?

Answer: Read the journals recommended throughout this text. When reading the newspaper, focus on these issues, which are written about every day. Talk to other PAs and get a sense for what's going on in this arena. How does it affect them?

"I feel that 'managed care' is an important concern at this time. Some providers feel that the insurance companies are now dictating how long a patient can remain in the hospital for a given illness. For example, until recently, mothers were allowed only one day in the hospital after having a baby, so-called drive-by deliveries. On the other hand, however, we must do something with respect to excessive health care costs. It's a real dilemma."

MOTIVATION TO BECOME A PA

Question: Why do you want to be a PA?

In other words: Have you thought intelligently about why you want to be a PA?

Answer: You must answer this question in 250 words or less and provide an answer that shows insight and enthusiasm:

> After serving as a hospital corpsman for four years and an emergency room technician for one year, I found a niche in health care. I enjoy providing comfort to patients and placing them at ease. I also enjoy being a member of the team and doing my part to provide the best quality of care to the patient.
>
> I want to do more, however. I would like to be able to diagnose and treat patients as well. Although I love my current job, I feel that I could contribute much more in this newly enhanced role as a PA.
>
> I have thought about medical school; I have a family and I do not have the time, nor the inclination, to spend the next eight or so years of my life pursuing that goal. From what I have experienced, PAs have a challenging and rewarding role in the health care system. I have never met a PA who disliked his or her job.
>
> I simply want to practice medicine. I like the fact that PAs have physicians available for consultation with difficult presentations. I feel no need to be independent, although I think in situations I'll be somewhat autonomous. This is why I prefer becoming a PA rather than a nurse-practitioner, who frequently practices independently.
>
> Finally, I like that PAs are trained in the medical model and can move from one specialty to the next without having to retrain. This is a benefit not even afforded the MD.

In less than 250 words, the applicant has managed to answer several questions and touch on several key points:

- Demonstrated experience
- Teamwork
- Enthusiasm
- Why he doesn't want to be an MD, nurse-practitioner, or nurse
- Understanding of dependent practitioner role
- Understanding of autonomy

Question: Have you applied to other programs?

In other words: How serious are you? Why have you chosen the programs you have? What's your logic in choosing the programs you have?

Answer: By applying to other programs, you show that you want to become a PA and are maximizing your chances of getting into school. In addition, you should be prepared to discuss why you selected the programs you have (your transcripts from various colleges frequently list other programs to which you've applied, so many times, the committee knows where else you've applied.)

- "I applied to Northeastern, Quinnipiac, and Duke because they offer a master's degree."
- "I applied to Yale, Quinnipiac, Northeastern, and Springfield College because my wife will be supporting me and our children, and if we have to move, she may not be able to find a job that pays enough to cover the rent and put food on the table."
- "I applied to Cornell, Alabama, and Cuyahoga because I'm really interested in doing surgery."

Question: What have you done to prepare yourself for this profession?

In other words: Are you a serious applicant or just testing the waters because you're not happy with your current profession?

Answer: Review your worksheets, and list all of your preparation and accomplishments to get you where you are:

> In addition to my degree in biology, I also worked as a nurse's aide for three years. Recently, I went back to night school to take courses in cell biology and pharmacology. In addition, I have volunteered at the local hospital's HIV clinic for the past six months. I have also shadowed two PAs this year; one works in internal medicine and the other works in OB-GYN. And, I have joined the AAPA and ConnAPA to keep up with current issues facing the profession.

Don't fabricate here. Hopefully, you have done something to prepare yourself for getting into PA school.

Question: Have you done anything to increase your chances of being accepted to the PA program?

In other words: This is especially important for reapplicants: Just how serious and committed are you? **What makes you stand out from the person sitting next to you this morning?**

Answer: This is your opportunity to shine. Tell the committee about all of the PAs you have contacted, shadowed, and communicated with. Tell them about the recent courses you've completed and all of your health care experience. Point out that you have joined your state Academy of Physician Assistants and the American Academy of Physician Assistants. Let them know, by name, any and all of their current students whom you have worked with. In other words, demonstrate that getting into PA school has been your mission for the past 12 months.

UNDERSTANDING OF THE PA PROFESSION

Question: What is your understanding of what PAs do?

In other words: Are you aware of the PA concept?

Answer: Do not recite the AAPA definition of a PA here. Personalize your answer based on your experience with PAs. If you have no experience with PAs, then don't try to fool the committee into thinking you do. They'll catch you. You may want to start with, "In my understanding . . ." Otherwise, give your understanding of the profession based on first-hand knowledge:

> Based on my experience as a technician in the emergency room, and through my recent shadowing of two PAs, I have observed several PAs in action. Most of them work autonomously but usually have the availability of a physician when needed. In the emergency room, the PAs are usually the first to see the patients when they arrive. They take a short history from the patient or Emergency Medical Technicians, perform a physical exam, and order the appropriate tests. At times, they suture, apply casts, or perform various other procedures.
>
> The internal medicine PAs are part of a team, working closely with other students, interns, residents, and the attending physician. They often round with the team and present and discuss their patients. They also report to the emergency room to interview their patients, write the History and Physical, order the appropriate tests, and formulate the initial plan.

This applicant is explaining, from personal experience, the role of the PA at her institution. This is much better than giving the AAPA definition of the profession, and, believe me, many people simply cite that definition instead of personalizing their answer.

Question: Tell us about the role you see the PA playing in the health care system.

In other words: Are you familiar with the PA concept?

Answer: This is similar to the foregoing question but with a little twist. Do not mention a hierarchy of physician, PA, nurse, and so on. Keep the focus on teamwork: "PAs are a part of the health care team, working with physicians, nurses, and other members to provide the best care to the patient."

Question: How do you feel about taking call or working 60 or more hours per week as a second-year student?

In other words: Do you know what you're getting yourself into?

Answer: You may be thinking, "But I thought PAs didn't have to work like interns, putting in so many hours." Although you may choose not to work so many hours as a PA, when you are a PA student and on rotation, you are expected to work as many hours as medical students or interns. The correct response would be, "I'm prepared to do whatever it takes to be a PA. I have spoken with several PA students, and I know what I am up against. I welcome the challenge of learning all that I can while I'm in school."

INTERPERSONAL SKILLS AND BEHAVIOR

Question: Describe an interaction you have had with a patient that made an impact on you.

In other words: Do you have compassion or are you simply science oriented, more interested in the pathology than the patient?

Answer: Be prepared to discuss a patient who has made an impact on you in some way. Let the committee know what the situation was, how the patient made out, and what you've learned from him or her.

My first trauma patient was a 23-year-old Portuguese gentleman who was involved in an industrial fire. He spoke no English. I remember the burn team coming to the emergency room and assessing him. He appeared to be in no pain, even though he was burned over most of his body. I originally thought he was wearing gloves, until someone pointed out that what I saw was his skin hanging from his hands.

The burn team assessed the patient, left the room, and began drawing figures on a piece of paper. They concluded that the man had less than a 3% chance of surviving. They went back into the trauma room, this time with an interpreter, and explained the situation to the patient. They asked him if he wanted them to operate, which would be extremely painful, or simply make him comfortable. I remember his response was to operate. "What else would a 23-year-old say," I thought?

The patient died after surgery, but I will never forget him, and how he must have felt lying on the trauma room table, not understanding English, and having someone ask if he preferred to live in pain or die.

Question: What do you think is the most difficult situation described in the interview scenarios that you completed earlier today? Why?

In other words: Do you have any hidden feelings about AIDS patients, psychiatric patients, or drug addicts?

Answer: Don't shoot yourself in the foot. Hopefully, you did not give any controversial answers. You can simply reply, in response to the trauma patient with HIV: "Every day I witness staff members in the hospital not taking universal precautions by wearing gloves or protective eyewear. I do my best to lead by example and always protect myself, but I must admit that I cringe when I see others take universal precautions so lightly." This response shifts the focus off the HIV-positive patient and concentrates on the issue of universal precautions.

ABILITY TO HANDLE STRESS

Question: Describe the most stressful work or academic situation you have been in, and tell us how you dealt with it.

In other words: What constitutes stress to you, and do you know how to cope with stress?

Answer: The committee knows that interviewing for PA school is stressful enough, and committee members probably have a good idea of your ability to handle it at this point. But give them a little more insight by example:

> I find the best way to deal with stress is to avoid it! But that isn't always possible. My most stressful situation came as a junior officer in the Air Force. I was placed in charge of a bomb cleanup operation at Nellis Air Force base in Nevada. I had 40 people working for me—carpenters, explosive ordnance disposal people, and several truck drivers. The range we were cleaning was used by F-16 pilots to practice bombing skills. We had to sweep the range, remove the live ordnance that remained, and build new targets. Under each old piece of plywood we found a rattlesnake. Between the bombs and the snakes, I was never so scared in my life; and I was in charge!
>
> To get through the situation, I relied on the senior noncommissioned officers from each group. Each morning we'd meet and make a plan of action. We kept in contact via radio all day. I'm proud to say that we had no casualties, and we all received a letter of commendation from our commanding officer. Teamwork got us through.

Although this is a dramatic story, for which many people have no similar experience, the applicant explained that he relied on others' help to get everyone through the situation. He used teamwork and planning each day to get through.

By the way, providing a copy of a letter of commendation in your application will provide verification for your statement.

Question: How do you usually deal with stress?

In other words: Do you have any stress-relieving activities? Some interviewers may also ask this question to see if you exercise.

Answer: I recommend that you take up some form of exercise for your own good. Then you can answer, "I run three miles a day or I do yoga five times per week."

Question: What kind of personal stress do you see associated with our PA program?

In other words: Do you have a realistic view of the rigor of the program? Do you have any hidden fears about coming here to school?

Answer: "After speaking to several of your students, both first year and second year, I am aware of how difficult the two years will be. For instance, I know that the didactic phase is extremely comprehensive and fast paced. In addition, I'm aware of the amount of hours I'll be expected to put in on clinical rotations. However, I am confident that my previous college work in chemistry and biology has prepared me well for further study, and I have never been afraid to roll up my sleeves and work long, hard hours. I look forward to the challenge."

Question: What kind of stress do you see associated with the PA profession?

In other words: Are you aware of how far the profession has come, and what challenges still lie ahead?

Answer: "The PA profession has come a long way in a short time. I know that the early PAs had to fight for all of the respect and privileges that everyone enjoys today. However, there are still issues to be resolved and more work to be done. Some nurses and nurse-practitioners take issue with the scope of PA practice—a case in point is Mississippi. We will always face new challenges, especially with health care reform, but the profession has come too far, and if PAs continue doing as well as they have done in the past, the profession will continue to grow."

PERSONAL CHARACTERISTICS

Question: What do you do outside of work or academic studies?

In other words: Are you a well-rounded person?

Answer: Go back to your worksheets in Chapter 6 and make a list of your extracurricular activities. List things you like to do: biking, hiking, running, investing, playing in a band, and so on.

Question: Please discuss your answer to question no. X on the interview questionnaire. What did you mean by X on your essay?

In other words: Can you think on your feet?

Answer: As mentioned already, the best way to deal with stress is to avoid it. Don't write anything controversial on your questionnaire or narrative and you'll never have to answer a question like this. But if you do, keep your cool, take a deep breath, and answer the question to the best of your ability. Don't add insult to injury by arguing your point. Perhaps you misunderstood the original question.

Question: Your file indicates that you have had difficulty with X (e.g., time management, science coursework). Would you like to explain this?

In other words: Have you thought about your shortcomings? What have you done to change things?

Answer: Of course, you would like to comment. You have hopefully anticipated this question about your grades or why you flunked freshman chemistry in college. "In high school I had no real focus in life and I simply wanted to graduate. After working for Dr. Smith and realizing I loved medicine, I went to college with a purpose, to get into PA school, and my grades improved tremendously."

Question: What accommodations, if any, do you need to successfully complete this program?

In other words: Is there any part of the program you will not participate in?

Answer: We had several women in our class who weren't thrilled with the idea of classmates doing breast exams on one another. This issue came up at the beginning of our physical exam sessions. It caused a lot of stress for the class and the students involved. If you feel strongly about an issue, with respect to the program, discuss it before you begin the program, but not necessarily at the interview.

MORE INTERVIEW QUESTIONS

The following questions may be similar to the foregoing ones. Keep in mind that specific examples and vignettes make for better answers than a simple yes or no. By the same token, keep your answers concise.

Question: So, tell us a little about yourself.

In other words: Why are you here?

Answer: Dig out those worksheets and compile a brief summary of your accomplishments. In 250 words or less, cover the following points (note that all of your answers do not have to be medically oriented):

1. Your strongest skills
2. Specific areas of knowledge
3. Greatest personality strengths
4. What you do best
5. Key accomplishments

Question: You have had several jobs in the past; how do we know you will finish the program if we accept you?

In other words: Do you have commitment and staying power?

Answer: This should be a two-part answer:

1. If it's true, admit to having moved around a bit. (It's obvious from your application.)
2. Convince the committee that you've seen the light, if you will, and tell them what specific steps you've taken to achieve your goal.

Question: Why do you think X school turned you down?

In other words: Did you take the time to find out why that school didn't accept you?

Answer: If you interviewed elsewhere or if you've been turned down for any reason, be sure to follow up on how you can improve your application. The program will usually tell you why you came up short. For example, "I was told that although I was a good applicant, the pool was so competitive this year that not all good candidates could feasibly be accepted. They told me to continue with my current medical experience."

Question: What are your strengths as an applicant?

In other words: Convince us that you are the right person for us.

Answer: You've probably already answered a similar question. Be sure to toot your own horn without being too cocky. Review your worksheets for all of the information you'll need on this one.

Question: What are your biggest weaknesses as an applicant, and what do you plan to do to correct them?

In other words: Please tell us that you don't walk on water, too.

Answer: They may be handing you a rope here, but you don't have to hang yourself. Everyone has weaknesses, but for an interview, you want to stay focused on the positive. Achieve a compromise: "I tend to work too many hours lately, but I realize how important my free time is, and I'm much happier when I get to do the things I love outside of work."

Question: Do you manage your time well?

In other words: Can you handle a program as difficult as this one? Will you require constant help?

Answer: "Yes, I can. I have a set of written goals, and I prioritize my time so as to accomplish them all in the order of their importance, and in a timely manner." (I already told you having written goals is important!)

Question: Do you prefer to work with others or by yourself?

In other words: How do you get along with your coworkers?

Answer: "I get along very well with others. I usually reach out to people, or I can simply hold your hand and be a friend in time of need. I consider myself to be a team player."

Question: Your supervising MD tells you to do something that you know is dead wrong; what do you do?

In other words: How's your judgment?

Answer: "I certainly do not know what it is like to be a PA in that situation, but it seems that I would have to bring the possible error to his or her attention, tactfully, and be sure that it gets resolved." A little humility goes a long way.

Question: What interests you most about our school?

In other words: Have you done your homework?

Answer: This is a very personal choice; just be prepared for the question and answer it to the best of your ability. Let the committee know that you have specific reasons for being interested in the school.

Question: What would be your ideal job as a PA?

In other words: Are you open-minded?

Answer: The key here is to show that you have an open mind, yet don't try to deceive the committee. If all of your experience is in orthopedics, don't try to tell the committee that you've always wanted to work in an HIV clinic. Give a well-balanced answer:

> Although I feel my current interest is in orthopedics, I have never worked in any other area. I know from talking with several of your graduate students that they came into the program with certain inclinations; but after doing a rotation in another specialty, they liked it enough to work in that area after graduation. I will try to keep an open mind.

Question: What did you learn from your overseas internship or experience?

In other words: What did you learn from your overseas internship or experience?

Answer: That's right, this question is as straightforward as they come, yet too many applicants blow it. Think about your travel overseas, and be prepared to discuss the impact it had on you. Did you take advantage of the local culture? Did you mix with the locals? Did you make any lasting friendships? You didn't blow the opportunity, did you?

Question: What do you want to be doing five years from now?

In other words: Do you have any goals?

Answer: Of course, you have goals. I won't comment much more here other than to say that I hope you still want to be a PA in five years and that you'll still want to contribute to the medical community in a positive way. (Note: If you haven't filled out your goal sheet yet, do so now!)

Question: Have you ever seen anyone die?

In other words: Are you prepared to deal with death?

Answer: This was a favorite question of one of our committee members, usually before the applicant sat down. If you have never seen anyone die, that's OK. You are not expected to know what it is like to be a PA. If you have seen someone die, reflect on the situation with empathy and explain that you are capable of carrying on. Death is a part of life. Don't answer, as one applicant did, "Of course, I've seen people die. I was in a gang."

INNOCENT QUESTIONS?

There are no innocent questions. Remember, you are being evaluated from the time you walk into the building until the time you leave at the end of the day.

Question: What is your opinion of the health care reform bill that is currently moving through Congress?

In other words: Do you have an opinion about the health care rights of individuals?

Answer: With hot topics in current events or politics, try to respond to the main concept or principle without getting involved in a political discussion. On health care reform, you might say, "I believe that every American has a right to access health care, but how that should happen is controversial. I couldn't claim to know enough to make a judgment about the proposals."

Question: How are you today?

In other words: Are you a positive or negative person?

Answer: "I'm fine, thank you." That's all that is required. Do not go on about the parking lot being full, or the terrible night's sleep you had, or how nervous you are.

Question: Did you have any trouble finding us?

In other words: Did you use the resources available to you?

Answer: "No trouble at all; I called the office ahead of time for directions."

Question: What was the last movie you saw?

In other words: What are you interested in?

Answer: I can't tell you what kind of movies to go see. Personally, I'm into horror movies, but I wouldn't tell the admission's committee that. An Oscar winner is always a safe bet.

Question: What was the most difficult question that you were asked in X interview (at another PA program)?

In other words: Have you thought about that interview?

Answer: Tell the committee that you were well prepared for the interview, and they did not ask you any questions that you did not anticipate.

CLOSING THE INTERVIEW

Question: What will you do if you don't get in this year?

In other words: Will you give up?

Answer: In Appendix A, I cover specific steps to take if you do not get in this year. Do not read too much into the question. Many interviewers ask this of everyone and want to know whether you will apply again.

Your response? "I will consult with the program director, find out why I was not accepted, and strive to accomplish those things for next year."

Question: Do you have any questions for us? (We discussed this question and the answer to it in the previous chapter.)

Finally, it is worth repeating that you should not use these same answers at the interview. Study your worksheets and spend some time compiling your own answers to questions. Be honest and genuine. Remember, what's the worst thing that can happen?

[CHAPTER 10]

Financial Aid

THE ALL-IMPORTANT QUESTION

Can I afford to go to PA school? The question you should be asking is this: **Can I afford not to go to PA school?** If your goal is to become a PA, then the answer to that question is easy. The worst thing you can do is shy away from applying because you think you won't be able to afford it and then live the rest of your life wondering, "What if?"

Can I Afford not to Go to PA School?

When I applied to Yale and spoke to students at the open house, they told me that if I was accepted, the program would do its best to ensure that I got through financially. They were right. I may have borrowed a little more than I intended, but the money was available. As you will soon find out, there are plenty of opportunities for loans, grants, scholarships, and so on. It does, however, take a little work on your part. But because you have set your goals and you're focused, you are prepared for anything.

The following chapter is not meant to be a step-by-step guide for filling out financial aid forms. The focus of this book, remember, is getting into the PA school of your choice. The purpose of this chapter is to give you some valuable resources and advice on finding financial aid.

THE PLAN OF ACTION

I can still remember the butterflies I felt in my stomach when I sent my deposit in to Yale. Reality set in: "I'm going to PA school." Immediately, the thoughts began racing in my head: "I'm giving up my annual salary, plus I'm paying close to $14,000 per year for tuition, plus I'm borrowing money for living expenses and to support my family." I began doing the math and doubt started to slowly creep in. However, I quickly remembered my goals and how hard I had worked to get that far. I needed to stay the course and focus.

I knew somehow that everything would work out for the best. I don't regret one minute of my decision. In fact, I'm happier than I ever thought I would be. I also fully recovered from the financial strain. Here's how.

Budget

We've all heard the word *budget* before and have probably tried to write down our income on one side of a piece of paper and our expenses on the other. The problem is that we usually have many more expenses than we're willing to write down. **The only effective way to properly attempt a budget is to write down every penny you spend for at least one month.** Everything counts, from dinner to clothes to a can of Coke. If you're married, your spouse will have to participate, too. After 30 days, count how much you spend and compare it with your original calculations. I think you'll be shocked at how much more you actually spend. But don't worry; now you can realistically see where all of your money is going and figure out ways to cut the fat.

To prepare you for some of the expenses that you'll encounter when attending PA school, I've included a list of items that you'll most likely have to spend money on:

- Rent or mortgage
- Groceries
- Utilities, including Internet
- Telephones
- Clothes
- Laundry and dry cleaning
- Entertainment
- Personal expenses
- Transportation
- Books
- Travel

- Insurance
- Medical
- Medical equipment (e.g., stethoscope, otoscope)
- Child care
- Credit cards
- Tuition
- Fees
- Parking
- Miscellaneous

Explore your Options

The biggest mistake I made in PA school, now that I look back on it, was quitting my part-time job. Every program will tell you that you can't work while in PA school. You get so worked up about finally getting accepted that you absolutely want to do your best. You think that by not working you will be able to concentrate more on school. The problem is, if you're flat broke at the end of the semester, and your next financial aid check is still weeks away, you won't be able to concentrate too well anyway. You might as well work. I gave up a part-time job that paid about $300 per week. Do some quick math—that's more than $15,000 per year. Ouch!

In contrast, if you really don't need the money, then don't work. It will be especially hard to keep a job once you start clinical rotations. This is definitely a personal choice. All I'm trying to say is use your own judgment; every program will advise you against working, but ultimately you have to make the decision that's best for you.

NEED-BASED AID

You will hear the term *need-based aid* a lot once you begin filling out the vast number of financial aid forms. Need-based aid is available to help you finance your PA education. Because you and your family are expected to contribute to the cost of this education, this aid is supplementary. Here is the formula programs use to determine whether you qualify for need-based aid:

Cost of attendance − student contribution = student financial need

As I mentioned already, once I was accepted to Yale, the program assured me that I would have every opportunity to complete the program, regardless of my ability to pay. This, in fact, is the underlying philosophy of need-based aid:

- Access to a program that best suits your needs
- Persistence, in that the inability to pay should not prevent you from finishing school
- Fairness, in that your family contribution will be determined fairly.

Who is an Independent Student?

Until July 23, 1992, all graduate students were considered independent, for federal aid purposes, if they were older than 24 or younger than 24 and not claimed as a dependent on anyone's income tax statement for the first calendar year in which they were seeking aid.

However, most schools ask for parental information even if you are totally independent and left the nest 20 years ago. You will be asked to obtain your parents' tax returns and pertinent financial information.

I personally did not ask my mom for her information, and because I did not submit any of her financial records, I left myself at risk of not receiving certain funds. In other words, if there was money left over after all other students who did submit parental information were taken care of, then I could receive that same aid.

HOW IS NEED DETERMINED?

Most PA programs should provide you with a budget worksheet that you can use to determine your cost of attendance for that institution.

Need Analysis

Your financial contribution is based on a congressional formula called congressional methodology (CM). Need analysis is a process used to estimate how much you will need of the congressional methodology to supplement your theoretically available resources. The two components include cost of attendance and an estimate of your family's ability to contribute.

Congressional methodology: Congressional methodology uses taxable and nontaxable base-year income to calculate the expected student contribution.

Student contribution: The student contribution (SC) is the amount you and your spouse are expected to contribute to finance your education. This amount is the same for all schools. Once this figure is determined, it is subtracted from the cost of attendance, and the remaining amount is your financial need.

The resources used to calculate the SC include items like savings, school-year earnings, and spousal income. Your expected contribution is based on an analysis of your income and asset information, size of household, and number of family members in college.

Students are expected to contribute 35% of their assets each year to meet educational needs.

Parental contribution: The parental contribution includes calculations based on parental income, expenses, and assets. Income includes items like social security, welfare, and dividends, as well as job salaries.

Professional Judgment

About now you may be asking, "Does anyone, besides a computer, ever look at my financial information and make a personal decision based on my circumstances?" The answer is yes. The financial aid counselor knows that even though you made $30,000 last year, you will lose some or all of that income this year. Counselors will use their professional judgment when allowing or disallowing certain funds. Needless to say, make friends with someone in the financial aid office quickly.

ORGANIZE YOUR FINANCIAL RECORDS

Suggestions

1. Follow instructions on every form.
2. Copy all forms.
3. Keep separate folders for each school.
4. Keep copies of at least two years of tax returns.

5. Gather all account numbers on bank statements, stocks, mutual funds, and so on.

6. Obtain all signatures from parents, spouse, and so on.

7. Put your name and Social Security number on all pages.

8. Respond immediately to all requests from lenders.

9. Follow up on everything.

10. Report any change in status immediately.

FEDERAL FINANCIAL AID

Before reading about federal financial aid, please remember that program rules sometimes change and that new financial aid options may occur at any time. Be sure to check http://studentaid.ed.gov for updated information.

As part of the Higher Education Act, to qualify for federal financial aid, you must meet the following requirements:

1. Be enrolled as a student in a specific program.

2. Be a U.S. citizen or eligible noncitizen.

3. Be making satisfactory progress in your course of study.

4. Neither be in default nor owe a refund for any federal aid received in the past.

5. Be enrolled at least half-time (6 semester hours).

6. Have a valid Social Security number (unless you are from the Republic of the Marshall Islands, the Federated States of Micronesia, or the Republic of Palau).

7. Be registered with the Selective Service if you are male and 18 to 25 years of age.

8. Not have a drug conviction for an offense that occurred while you were receiving federal student aid (e.g., grants, loans, work-study)

9. Be able to demonstrate financial need.

Address any questions you have to the Federal Student Aid Information Center Hotline (1-800-4-FED-AID, or TDD 1-800-369-0518). You can call the hotline to check on which schools participate in federal aid, eligibility requirements, how awards are determined, complaints, and the verification process and to order publications.

Federal Perkins Loan

The federal Perkins loan, currently at 5% interest, is available to under-graduate and graduate students. If you apply for this loan, you receive the money from your individual school rather than from the bank. You can borrow up to $6,000 per year for a maximum of $60,000 (including undergraduate loans). To qualify for the Perkins loan, you must demon-strate financial need, as determined by your financial aid application. This is the loan that you may not receive if you fail to include your parents' financial information with your application.

Sample Repayment Table for Federal Perkins Loan

Total Indebtedness	Number of Payments	Monthly Payment	Total Interest Charges	Total Repaid
$4,500	120	$47.73	$1,227.60	$5,727.60
9,000	120	95.46	2,455.20	11,455.20
18,000	120	190.92	4,910.40	22,910.40

Source: U.S. Department of Education

Federal Stafford Student Loan Program

Stafford loans are offered through your bank, credit union, or other lend-ing institutions. There are two types: subsidized and unsubsidized To qual-ify for a Stafford loan, you must demonstrate financial need, as determined by the CM formula. The interest rate varies. Stafford loans are based on need, not creditworthiness. Therefore, no cosigner is necessary.

Subsidized direct or FFEL Stafford loans: Graduate students may borrow between $3,500 and $8,500 per year depending upon grade level.

Unsubsidized direct or FFEL Stafford loans: Students may bor-row between $5,500 and $20,500 per year depending on grade and dependency status.

Direct Stafford loans: Same as the above two but funded by the U.S. Department of Education.

Sample Repayment Table for Stafford Loan (8% interest)

Loan Amount	No. of Months to Pay in Full					
	60	72	84	96	108	120
$1,000	20.28	17.54	15.59	14.14	13.02	12.14
5,000	101.39	87.67	77.94	70.69	65.10	60.67
6,000	121.66	105.20	93.52	84.83	78.12	72.80
6,500	131.80	113.97	101.32	91.90	84.63	78.87
7,500	152.08	131.50	116.90	106.03	97.65	91.00

Source: U.S. Department of Education

Direct and FFEL Plus Loans for Graduate and Professional Students

Direct and FFEL Plus loans are for students with a good credit history. The maximum amount is the cost of attendance less any other financial aid received. The current interest rate for the direct loan program is 7.9%. The current interest rate for the FFEL is 8.5%.

Sample Repayment Table for Direct Loan (7.9% Interest)

Loan Amount	No. of Months to Pay in Full					
	60	72	84	96	108	120
$1,000	20.23	17.48	15.54	14.09	12.97	12.08
5,000	101.14	87.42	77.68	70.43	64.83	60.40
6,000	121.37	104.91	93.22	84.52	77.80	72.48
6,500	131.49	113.65	100.99	91.56	84.29	78.52
7,500	151.71	131.13	116.52	105.64	97.25	90.60

Sample Repayment Table for FFEL Plus (8.5% Interest)

Loan Amount	No. of Months to Pay in Full					
	60	72	84	96	108	120
$1,000	20.52	17.78	15.84	14.39	13.28	12.40
5,000	102.58	88.89	79.18	71.96	66.40	61.99
6,000	123.10	106.67	95.02	86.35	79.68	74.39
6,500	133.36	115.56	102.94	93.55	86.32	80.59
7,500	153.87	133.34	118.77	107.94	99.60	92.99

Student Loan Comparison Chart

Loan Program	Eligibility	Award Amounts	Interest Rates	Lender/Length of Repayment
Federal Perkins Loans	Undergraduate and graduate students	Undergraduate—up to $5,500 a year (maximum of $27,500 as an undergraduate) Graduate—up to $8,000 a year (maximum of $60,000, including undergraduate loans) Amount actually received depends on financial need, amount of other aid, availability of funds at school	5%	Lender is your school Repay your school or its agent Up to 10 years to repay, depending on amount owed

(Continued)

Student Loan Comparison Chart (*Continued*)

Loan Program	Eligibility	Award Amounts	Interest Rates	Lender/Length of Repayment
FFEL Stafford Loans— subsidized and unsubsidized	Undergraduate and graduate students; must be enrolled at least half-time	Depends on grade level in school and dependency status (see "Maximum Annual Loan Limits Chart—Subsidized and Unsubsidized Direct and FFEL Stafford Loans" chart) Financial need is required for subsidized loans Financial need not necessary for unsubsidized loans	Fixed rate of 6.0% for subsidized loans and 6.8% for unsubsidized loans made to undergraduate students Graduate students have a 6.8% fixed interest rate The federal government pays interest on subsidized loans during school and certain other periods The borrower pays all interest on unsubsidized loans	Lender is a bank, credit union, or other participating private lender Repay the loan holder or its agent Between 10 and 25 years to repay, depending on amount owed and type of repayment plan selected
FFEL PLUS Loans	Parents of dependent undergraduate students enrolled at least half-time (see dependency status) Graduate or professional degree students enrolled at least half-time Borrower must not have negative credit history	Student's cost of attendance – other aid student receives = maximum loan amount	Fixed rate at 8.5% for loans first disbursed on or after July 1, 2006; borrower pays all interest	Same as for FFEL Stafford Loans above
Direct PLUS Loans	Same as above	Same as above	Fixed rate at 7.9% for loans first disbursed on or after July 1, 2006; borrower pays all interest	Same as for direct Stafford loans above, except that income-contingent repayment plan is not an option

FEDERAL GRANT PROGRAMS

National Health Service Corps (NHSC)

An excellent program, the National Health Service Corps covers tuition and provides you with a monthly stipend. You will incur a two-year obligation to a designated (underserved) location. You will be given several sites to select from throughout the country. You will be required to contact those sites for availability and negotiate a salary. Four hundred awards are given out per year. You must fill out a questionnaire and an application to be considered for an award.

Contact: NHSC Scholarships
Division of Applications and Awards
5600 Fishers Lane, Room 8A-55

Rockville, Maryland, 20857
(301) 594-4400

http://www.hrsa.gov

Indian Health Service (IHS)

The Indian Health Service requires a minimum two-year obligation for two years of financial support. Priority is given to Native American students, but others may apply.

Contact the IHS Scholarship Office at (800) 962-2817 or via the web at http://www.ihs.gov

Department of Health and Human Services Scholarships for Health Profession Students from Disadvantaged Backgrounds

This program is designed to assist health professional students and practitioners from disadvantaged backgrounds. Applicants must be able to prove financial need and prove enrollment or acceptance for enrollment to a program. They must also be full-time students. Visit http://www.federalgrantswire.com/scholarships-for-health-professionals.

State Programs

State programs include loan forgiveness, for which you can work at a designated clinic or site in an underserved area and receive up to $20,000 in loan forgiveness. Another good program is the Health Profession Shortage Area (HPSA) program, which provides loans at a dollar-for-dollar match for educational loans.

Contact the NHSC at (877) 313-1823 or (301) 446-1630 (in the Washington, D.C., area), or visit http://nhsc.hrsa.gov/.

AAPA Constituent Chapters

Most of the state chapters of the AAPA offer some sort of scholarship program for students. Contact your state chapter for availability (Appendix E).

Estimated PA Program Tuition and Costs (ARC-PA. www.arc-pa.org)

State		Program Length (Months)	Resident Tuition	Non-resident TuitionT[3]	Financial Aid Available
AL	University of Alabama at Birmingham	27	$28,560	$70,800	Yes
AL	University of South Alabama	27	$32,000	$63,000	Yes
AR	Harding University	28	$54,320	$54,320	Yes
AZ	Arizona School of Health Sciences	26	$50,060	$50,060	Yes
AZ	Midwestern University, Glendale	27	$68,373	$68,373	Yes
CA	Charles Drew University of Medicine and Science	24	$28,000	$28,000	Yes
CA	Keck School of Medicine of the University of Southern California	33	$111,342	$111,342	Yes
CA	Loma Linda University	24	$70,000	$70,000	Yes
CA	Riverside Community College	24	$2,314	$17,444	Yes
CA	Samuel Merritt College	28	$78,465	$78,465	Yes
CA	San Joaquin Valley College	24	$46,950	$46,950	Yes
CA	Stanford University	16	$29,445	$38,445	Yes
CA	Touro University, California	32	$78,000	$78,000	Yes
CA	University of California, Davis	24	$23,198	$39,424	Yes
CA	Western University of Health Sciences	24	$56,000	$56,000	Yes

(Continued)

Estimated PA Program Tuition and Costs (ARC-PA. www.arc-pa.org) (*Continued*)

State		Program Length (Months)	Resident Tuition	Non-resident TuitionT[3]	Financial Aid Available
CO	Red Rocks Community College	24	$32,000	$42,000	Yes
CO	University of Colorado Denver, Anschutz Medical Campus	36	$37,840	$75,320	Yes
CT	Quinnipiac University	27	$69,170	$69,170	Yes
CT	Yale University	27	$65,000	$65,000	Yes
DC	George Washington University	24	$67,000	$67,000	Yes
DC	George Washington University[4,5]	36	$90,000	$90,000	Yes
DC	Howard University	26	$35,050	$35,050	Yes
FL	Barry University	28	$55,046	$55,046	Yes
FL	Miami Dade College	22	$19,262	$27,953	Yes
FL	Nova Southeastern University, Fort Lauderdale	27	$52,360	$54,063	Yes
FL	Nova Southeastern University, Naples	27	$52,360	$54,063	Yes
FL	Nova Southeastern University, Orlando	27	$55,510	$56,770	Yes
FL	University of Florida	24	$27,303	$52,510	Yes
GA	Emory University	28	$53,900	$53,900	Yes
GA	Medical College of Georgia	27	$31,500	$63,588	Yes
GA	Mercer University	28	$50,351	$50,351	Yes

(*Continued*)

Estimated PA Program Tuition and Costs (ARC-PA. www.arc-pa.org) (*Continued*)

State		Program Length (Months)	Resident Tuition	Non-resident TuitionT[3]	Financial Aid Available
GA	South University	27	$58,050	$58,050	Yes
IA	Des Moines University	25	$48,000	$48,000	Yes
IA	University of Iowa	25	$28,890	$66,000	Yes
ID	Idaho State University	24	$49,725	$81,085	Yes
IL	John H. Stroger Jr. Hospital of Cook County/Malcolm X College	25	$6,250	$18,000	Yes
IL	Midwestern University-Downers Grove	27	$63,780	$63,780	Yes
IL	Rosalind Franklin University of Medicine and Science	24	$48,124	$48,124	Yes
IL	Southern Illinois University, Carbondale	26	$51,920	$77,880	Yes
IN	Butler University	30	$79,230	$79,230	Yes
IN	University of Saint Francis	27	$68,000	$68,000	Yes
KS	Wichita State University	26	$20,085	$50,212	Yes
KY	University of Kentucky	32	$31,255	$66,430	Yes
LA	Louisiana State University Health Sciences Center	27	$12,000	$18,000	Yes
MA	Massachusetts College of Pharmacy and Health Sciences, Boston	30	$88,350	$88,350	Yes

(*Continued*)

Estimated PA Program Tuition and Costs (ARC-PA. www.arc-pa.org) (*Continued*)

State		Program Length (Months)	Resident Tuition	Non-resident TuitionT[3]	Financial Aid Available
MA	Massachusetts College of Pharmacy and Health Sciences, Worcester[4]	24	$64,000	$64,000	Yes
MA	Northeastern University	24	$49,620	$49,620	Yes
MA	Springfield College	27	$86,280	$86,280	Yes
MA	Springfield College[4,5]	63	$24,075	$24,075	Yes
MD	Anne Arundel Community College	25	$19,024	$39,830	Yes
MD	Towson University CCBC Essex	26	$20,000	$38,000	Yes
MD	University of Maryland, Eastern Shore	24	$18,930	$36,519	Yes
ME	University of New England	24	$64,000	$64,000	Yes
MI	Central Michigan University	27	$43,920	$81,360	Yes
MI	Grand Valley State University	28	$37,885	$62,040	Yes
MI	University of Detroit Mercy	24	$64,170	$64,170	Yes
MI	Wayne State University	24	$26,000	$41,000	Yes
MI	Western Michigan University	24	$32,584	$45,855	Yes
MN	Augsburg College	36	$67,000	$67,000	Yes
MO	Missouri State University	24	$16,517	$32,704	Yes
MO	Saint Louis University	27	$64,395	$64,395	Yes

(*Continued*)

Estimated PA Program Tuition and Costs (ARC-PA. www.arc-pa.org) (*Continued*)

State		Program Length (Months)	Resident Tuition	Non-resident TuitionT[3]	Financial Aid Available
MT	Rocky Mountain College	26	$57,000	$57,000	Yes
NC	Duke University	24	$55,686	$55,686	Yes
NC	East Carolina University	27	$18,000	$54,842	Yes
NC	Methodist University	28	$50,000	$50,000	Yes
NC	Wake Forest University	24	$45,476	$45,476	Yes
NC	Wingate University	27	$56,000	$56,000	Yes
ND	University of North Dakota	24	$30,000	$30,000	Yes
NE	Union College	33	$68,500	$68,500	Yes
NE	University of Nebraska Medical Center	28	$29,212	$78,750	Yes
NH	Massachusetts College of Pharmacy and Health Sciences-Manchester	24	$64,000	$64,000	Yes
NJ	Seton Hall University	36	$84,000	$84,000	Yes
NJ	University of Medicine and Dentistry of New Jersey	36	$44,700	$67,050	Yes
NM	University of New Mexico	25	$15,789	$38,081	Yes
NM	University of St. Francis	27	$62,206	$62,206	Yes
NV	Touro University, Nevada	30	$57,000	$57,000	Yes
NY	Albany Medical College	28	$43,680	$43,680	Yes
NY	CUNY/Sophie Davis School of Biomedical Education	29	$12,380	$30,240	Yes

(*Continued*)

Estimated PA Program Tuition and Costs (ARC-PA. www.arc-pa.org) (Continued)

State		Program Length (Months)	Resident Tuition	Non-resident TuitionT[3]	Financial Aid Available
NY	Cornell University	26	$67272	$67272	Yes
NY	D'Youville College	36	$49,800	$49,800	Yes
NY	Daemen College	36	$78,660	$78,660	Yes
NY	Daemen College[4,5]	60	$75,000	$75,000	Yes
NY	Hofstra University	27	$49,200	$49,200	Yes
NY	Le Moyne College	24	$62,397	$62,397	Yes
NY	Long Island University	24	$56,000	$56,000	Yes
NY	Mercy College	27	$61,650	$61,650	Yes
NY	New York Institute of Technology	30	$76,734	$76,734	Yes
NY	Pace University, Lenox Hill Hospital	26	$76,000	$76,000	Yes
NY	Rochester Institute of Technology	48	$64,456	$64,456	Yes
NY	St. John's University	23	$47,500	$47,500	Yes
NY	State University of New York Downstate Medical Center	27	$16,212	$39,563	Yes
NY	Stony Brook University	24	$21,500	$33,200	Yes
NY	Touro College School of Health Sciences	23	$37,000	$37,000	Yes
NY	Touro College, Manhattan	32	$60,000	$60,000	Yes
NY	Touro College, Winthrop University Hospital[4]	23	$37,000	$37,000	Yes

(Continued)

Estimated PA Program Tuition and Costs (ARC-PA. www.arc-pa.org) (*Continued*)

State		Program Length (Months)	Resident Tuition	Non-resident TuitionT[3]	Financial Aid Available
NY	Wagner College	36	$81,900	$81,900	Yes
NY	Weill Cornell Medical College	26	$59,874	$59,874	Yes
NY	York College of the City University of New York	24	$11,500	$18,000	Yes
OH	Cuyahoga Community College	27	$23,000	$43,000	Yes
OH	Kettering College of Medical Arts	27	$57,820	$57,820	Yes
OH	Marietta College	27	$62,024	$62,024	Yes
OH	Mount Union College	27	$54,000	$54,000	Yes
OH	University of Findlay	27	$52,332	$52,332	Yes
OH	University of Toledo	27	$26,000	$40,000	Yes
OK	University of Oklahoma	30	$15,000	$45,000	Yes
OR	Oregon Health and Science University	26	$64,314	$64,314	Yes
OR	Pacific University	27	$60,780	$60,780	Yes
PA	Arcadia University	24	$54,000	$54,000	Yes
PA	Chatham University	24	$62,340	$62,340	Yes
PA	DeSales University	24	$58,240	$58,240	Yes
PA	DeSales University[4,5]	60	$123,400	$123,400	Yes
PA	Drexel University	27	$61,425	$61,425	Yes
PA	Duquesne University	27	$70,478	$70,478	Yes

(*Continued*)

Estimated PA Program Tuition and Costs (ARC-PA. www.arc-pa.org) (*Continued*)

State		Program Length (Months)	Resident Tuition	Non-resident TuitionT[3]	Financial Aid Available
PA	Gannon University	24	$40,000	$40,000	Yes
PA	Gannon University[4,5]	60	$40,000	$40,000	Yes
PA	King's College	24	$56,000	$56,000	Yes
PA	Lock Haven University of Pennsylvania	24	$28,294	$42,184	Yes
PA	Marywood University	27	$54,000	$54,000	Yes
PA	Pennsylvania College of Optometry	25	$54,500	$54,500	Yes
PA	Pennsylvania College of Technology	24	$34,450	$43,332	Yes
PA	Philadelphia College of Osteopathic Medicine	26	$55,526	$55,526	Yes
PA	Philadelphia University	25	$61,374	$61,374	Yes
PA	Saint Francis University	24	$69,170	$69,170	Yes
PA	Saint Francis University[4,5]	60	$138,254	$138,254	Yes
PA	Seton Hall University	27	$72,305	$72,305	Yes
SC	Medical University of South Carolina	27	$43,785	$87,297	Yes
SD	University of South Dakota	28	$24,934	$52,031	Yes
TN	South College	27	$63,772	$63,772	Yes
TN	Trevecca Nazarene University	27	$67,164	$67,164	Yes
TX	Baylor College of Medicine	30	$37,125	$37,125	Yes

(*Continued*)

Estimated PA Program Tuition and Costs (ARC-PA. www.arc-pa.org) (*Continued*)

State		Program Length (Months)	Resident Tuition	Non-resident TuitionT[3]	Financial Aid Available
TX	Interservice Physician Assistant Program	24	-	-	
TX	Texas Tech University Health Sciences Center	27	$22,525	$40,256	Yes
TX	University of North Texas Health Science Center at Fort Worth	34	$25,875	$66,185	Yes
TX	University of Texas Health Science Center at San Antonio	33	$19,840	$52,500	Yes
TX	University of Texas Medical Branch	26	$22,000	$55,200	Yes
TX	University of Texas, Pan American	28	$15,355	$39,447	Yes
TX	University of Texas Southwestern Medical Center	31	$21,600	$56,483	Yes
UT	University of Utah	27	$50,390	$75,029	Yes
VA	Eastern Virginia Medical School	27	$51,366	$53,935	Yes
VA	James Madison University	28	$24,620	$69,905	Yes
VA	Jefferson College of Health Sciences	27	$50,985	$50,985	Yes
VA	Shenandoah University	27	$55,610	$55,610	Yes
WA	University of Washington MEDEX	24	$42,992	$42,992	Yes
WI	Marquette University	32	$78,810	$78,810	Yes

(Continued)

Estimated PA Program Tuition and Costs (ARC-PA. www.arc-pa.org) (*Continued*)

State		Program Length (Months)	Resident Tuition	Non-resident TuitionT[3]	Financial Aid Available
WI	University of Wisconsin, LaCrosse; Gundersen; Mayo	24	$31,110	$71,550	Yes
WI	University of Wisconsin, Madison	24	$17,973	$59,598	Yes
WV	Mountain State University	34	$44,000	$44,000	Yes

Programs with Provisional Status

State		Program Length (Months)	Resident Tuition	Non-resident TuitionT[3]	Financial Aid Available
FL	Keiser University	24	$50,000	$50,000	Yes
NC	Wingate University	27	$58,800	$58,000	Yes
NH	Franklin Pierce University		$79,200	$79,200	Yes
NY	SUNY Upstate Medical Center	27	$19,532 (resident)	$20,788 (non-resident)	Yes
OH	Mount Union College	27	$54,000	$54,000	Yes
OK	University of Oklahoma, Tulsa	30	$30,000	$30,000	Yes
OK	University of Oklahoma, Tulsa	30	$30,000	$60,000	Yes
PA	University of Pittsburgh	27	$62,044 (resident)	$108,804 (non-resident)	Yes
TN	Bethel University	36	$60,000	$60,000	Yes
TN	Bethel College	27	$60,000	$60,000	Yes
TN	LIncoln Memorial	27	$77,091	$77,091	Yes

[CHAPTER 11]

The Internet for PA School Applicants

The Internet is a valuable resource for applicants to physician assistant school who want to research a particular PA program, gain more knowledge about the profession in general, or perhaps want to communicate with PAs and PA students online. In this chapter, I provide you with a number of Web sites that should prove valuable to you as an applicant.

Practically every PA program in the United States has a Web site that posts a variety of information relative to admission requirements, curriculum, student societies, tuition, financial aid, and student contacts. In addition, most PA program Web sites allow users to download a program brochure and application and to contact students who are currently attending the program.

The Internet also provides a variety of organizational and personal Web sites relative to the PA profession. Applicants can access these sites to learn more about current events facing the PA profession, and much more.

My personal Web site—www.andrewrodican.com (Getting into the Physician Assistant School of Your Choice)—is exclusively designed for PA school applicants and provide a variety of information relative to becoming a formidable candidate for PA school. Highlights of my site include:

- *PA links.* Find links to all of the previously mentioned Web sites.

- *Discussion group.* Join a PA school applicant discussion group. Learn from the experiences of other applicants who may have been through the application and interview process before.

- *FAQs.* Learn the answer to most of your questions relative to applying to PA school and the PA profession in general.

- *PA programs.* A complete listing of PA programs, with links to their Web sites.

- *Ask the author.* A forum in which users can e-mail directly with questions. I personally respond to all inquiries.

- *One-on-one coaching.* A personalized coaching service that allows the applicant to work exclusively with me on the application, essay, and interview.

- *Free e-newsletter.* Sign up for a free monthly e-newsletter that is e-mailed directly to you.

- *Financial aid.* Find out the latest news relevant to financial aid, with links to various Web sites.

- *Essay tip of the month.* Each month I publish a new tip for making your essay strong and persuasive.

WEBSITES

http://www.aapa.org (American Academy of Physician Assistants)

The American Academy of Physician Assistants (AAPA) is the only national organization that represents physician assistants in all specialties and employment settings. Membership includes physician assistants, physician assistant students, physician assistant hopefuls, and those interested in supporting the physician assistant profession. The AAPA Web site provides volumes of information. The following is a listing of resources available on the AAPA's web site:

- AAPA information
- PA organizations
- About PAs
- Member benefits and services
- CME and clinical issues
- Government issues
- Reimbursement issues
- Professional practice issues
- Employment and employer's guide
- Support the PA profession

http://www.paeaonline.org (Physician Assistant Education Association)

The Physician Assistant Education Association (PAEA) is the only national organization in the United States representing physician assistant (PA) educational programs.

http://appap.org (Association of Postgraduate Physician Assistant Programs)

The Association of Postgraduate Physician Assistant Programs (APPAP) provides educational, professional, and informational support to PAs.

http://www.jaapa.com/be core/j/index.jsp (Official Journal of the American Academy of Physician Assistants)

This is the official journal of the AAPA and is clinically oriented, geared toward practicing PAs and PA students. In addition to clinical articles, the journal frequently reports on issues relevant to the PA profession. The journal also provides a listing of employment opportunities.

http://www.caspaonline.org (Central Application Service for Physician Assistants)

The Central Application Service for Physician Assistants (CASPA) offers a Web-based application service that allows PA school applicants to apply to numerous participating educational programs by completing a single application.

www.fafsa.ed.gov (Federal Student Aid)

The Federal Student Aid Web site provides information relative to financial aid available from the U.S. Department of Education. The Federal student aid programs are the largest source of student aid in the United States, providing more than $60 billion a year in grants, loans, and work-study assistance. Here you'll find help for every stage of the financial aid process, whether you're in school or out of school.

http://www.arc-pa.org (Accreditation Review Commission on Education for the Physician Assistant)

The Accreditation Review Commission on Education for the Physician Assistant (ARC-PA) is the accrediting agency that protects the interests of the public and the PA profession by defining the standards for PA education and evaluating PA education programs in the territorial United States to ensure their compliance with those standards.

http://www.nccpa.net (National Commission of Certification of Physician Assistants)

The National Commission of Certification of Physician Assistants (NCCPA) is the only credentialing organization for physician assistants in the United States. Established as a not-for-profit organization in 1975, the NCCPA is dedicated to ensuring that certified physician assistants meet established standards of knowledge and clinical skills on entry into practice and throughout their careers. Every U.S. state, the District of Columbia, and the U.S. territories rely on NCCPA certification as a criterion for licensure or regulation of physician assistants. The NCCPA has certified approximately 60,000 physician assistants.

PA FORUMS ON THE INTERNET

This section covers a listing of PA forums available on the Internet. **By joining a forum, applicants can plug in to some of the hot topics facing the profession and get a sense for what PAs in general are thinking.** The applicant can also pose questions to the forum and perhaps locate PAs to shadow. Subscriptions are free, but you must be a subscriber to post to the forums. Once the server acknowledges your subscription, you can post to a list.

PA Professional Forum: PAs discussing general interest and non-clinical topics. Subscribe at http://physicianassistantforum.com/forums/forumdisplay.php?f=40; post messages to paforum@list.mc.duke.edu.

Physician Assistant Journal: See articles and reviews of PA literature as well as Continuing Medical Education (CME) offerings and potential jobs. Subscribe at http://jaapa.com.

The Internet is a valuable resource for PA school applicants. The applicant can learn volumes about the PA profession by visiting some of these key sites. In addition, it is possible to develop a rapport with PAs and PA students who may become mentors to you and who may also provide you with shadowing opportunities. Good luck with your search!

[CHAPTER 12]

PA Job Descriptions

This chapter is designed to introduce PA school applicants to the various clinical specialties and disciplines in which PAs practice. New specialties are emerging each year. In fact, the American Academy of Physician's Assistants (AAPA) notes that PAs practice in more than 60 different specialties. For more information on specialties, visit the AAPA's Web site at http://www.aapa.org.

In this chapter, I cover the seven areas of clinical medicine (family practice, emergency medicine, pediatrics, psychiatry, obstetrics and gynecology, internal medicine, and surgery) that many programs require as mandatory rotations (including *U.S. News and World Report's* top 10 PA schools).

Descriptions of each specialty include:

1. Description of duties
2. The team
3. Salary
4. Summary

The description of duties includes an account of the day-to-day activities and functions of a PA working in a given specialty. I point out the various clinical presentations and types of patients you can expect to evaluate and treat in that particular discipline, and I try to give you a sense of the physical and mental challenges associated with the job. For instance, some areas of medicine are more cerebral than others, whereas other specialties tend to be more task and procedure oriented.

After reading over the various job descriptions, you may come to some insightful conclusions. For instance, you may be surprised to find out that traditional family practice PAs don't necessarily get to spend a great deal of time with their patients, as reported in most of the PA literature. Many family practice PAs are so busy that they barely have time for lunch. You may be surprised to find out that surgery PAs actually have more of an opportunity to get to know patients and their families much better because they may have a patient on their service for several days.

I bring this up because the premise of this book is to set you apart from the competition. Many applicants come to the interview without a clue as to how real PAs function. They think PAs have unlimited time to spend with patients. It's refreshing, and it shows a great deal of insight, when an applicant is knowledgeable about the different jobs PAs perform and understands that what the literature says and what PAs actually do may be two different things.

During the course of interviews, 90% of applicants will say that they want to work in family practice or with AIDS patients. They think this is the politically correct answer. They fail to realize, however, that the people interviewing them are real PAs working in a variety of specialties. Fewer than 40% of all PAs work in family practice; that leaves more than 60% of all PAs to work in other areas—and PAs are needed in every specialty. I can't tell you how many applicants come to an interview with, for example, six years of orthopedic experience and then tell you they want to work in a totally different area. That may be a legitimate goal for some, but most are not being true to the committee, or themselves. **The key is to be consistent and to be honest. Don't fake it, because it won't work!**

The team consists of the professionals you will interact with the most on a daily basis. The PA profession is one that requires collaboration with a variety of medical and nonmedical personnel. The more you understand teamwork in the PA profession, the better off you'll be at interview time.

The salary is self-explanatory. I simply try to give you an idea of the earning potential of PAs in a variety of settings. Of course, salary varies depending on the type of practice (hospital versus clinic or private practice) and your negotiating skills.

The summary is a synopsis of the stress level, hours, educational opportunities, research opportunities, and job pace. The summary also gives you an idea of the type of person who tends to gravitate toward each specialty.

FAMILY PRACTICE

Description of Duties

Family practice is the cornerstone of the PA profession; approximately 40% of all PAs work in family practice. The family practice PA may work in a clinic (urban or rural) or for a private physician or group of physicians. For family practice, PAs generally require a strong breadth of knowledge in the following areas: pediatrics, internal medicine, dermatology, orthopedics, HIV/AIDS, cardiology, endocrinology, pulmonology, obstetrics and gynecology, and renal disease. In addition, the PA must develop the skills to perform minor surgery, splint and cast limbs, and remove foreign objects from the eyes, to name just a few.

The patients in a family practice setting are generally nonacute, except, perhaps, in a rural setting, where your practice may provide the only medical care for miles. Many patients are familiar to the practice and typically present with colds, flu, and minor ailments. Others, however, may present with more complex problems and require closer follow-up. Depending on the type and location of the practice, you may follow a great number of HIV and AIDS patients. You may also be required to go out into the community and provide care to the indigent population. In fact, many inner-city clinics cater specifically to this population.

In addition to the various acute illnesses evaluated and treated on a daily basis, there is also a very routine aspect to the job of family practice PA. For instance, family practice PAs perform numerous school, sports, and well-baby physical examinations. Many patients in the practice may be diabetic and/or hypertensive and require periodic, routine follow-up examinations. Administering immunizations is also an important part of the job.

Of course, like all specialties, the family practice PA works very closely with the supervising physician. Although the PA works fairly autonomously in this setting, the physician is always available for consultation on the more difficult cases.

Most family practice clinics have pharmacy, x-ray, and laboratory capabilities. Depending on the size and budget of the facility, the PA may be required to perform basic laboratory studies to confirm or rule out a diagnosis.

Contrary to popular belief (i.e., of many PA school applicants), a PA working in a family practice setting doesn't always have vast amounts of time to spend with patients. In fact, **many PAs in a busy family practice setting will see more than 40 patients per day, often skipping lunch to stay on schedule.** Generally, however, the hours are fairly regular, from 9 to 5, and there typically is no call or weekend duty.

The Team

The family practice team varies from office to office depending on the size of the practice. In general, PAs work alongside physicians, nurses, nurse-practitioners, medical assistants, and various clerical personnel. A larger practice may also employ x-ray technicians, laboratory technicians, and pharmacists.

Salary

Depending on the type of practice (solo, group, hospital clinic), family practice PAs earn in the middle of the salary range, from $68,000 to $85,000 per year. Of course, salary depends on the amount of clinical experience that you bring to the bargaining table. Some clinics are open during the evening hours and on weekends, which provides an opportunity for family practice PAs to earn an extra $3,000 to $10,000 per year in differential pay.

Summary

The family practice setting allows for a traditional role for PAs. The setting provides a great opportunity for PAs to enhance their clinical skills by evaluating and treating a variety of medical presentations. Although the job is not paced as leisurely as some may expect, the stress level is usually manageable, because the patients are nonacute. The job has the potential to become routine at times, but it is certainly not boring.

EMERGENCY MEDICINE

Description of Duties

About 8% of physician assistants work in the fast-paced arena of emergency medicine. Generally, an emergency room (ER) is divided into several sections: surgery, medicine, trauma, major medical, fast track, pediatrics, and psychiatry. Some PAs work in primarily one area, but many rotate through all areas depending on preference, experience, and hospital policy.

In the surgery section, patients usually have obvious complaints and injuries, and the role of PAs is highly oriented toward procedure; they do a lot of suturing, splinting and casting, removing foreign objects from the eyes, and wrapping sprains and strains. However, some patients may have more complex complaints, such as appendicitis, bowel obstruction, or kidney or gallstones, which involve further diagnostic work-up with x-rays and laboratory testing.

In the medicine section, PAs see a variety of common and complex patients with complaints of asthma, fever, shortness of breath, nausea and vomiting, dizziness, and so on. Many patients are elderly or have a history of diabetes or heart disease. Usually, PAs work closely with the patient's family physician, especially when the patient has a complicated past medical history. This area of the ER is less oriented toward tasks and procedures, and PAs are challenged to collect a thorough medical history and use excellent clinical skills to arrive at a diagnosis.

The trauma section of the ER is reserved for acute injuries sustained from, for example, motor vehicle accidents, gunshot wounds, falls, knife wounds, fights, ruptured aneurysms, and burns, to name a few. In this arena, PAs have a specific task as a member of the trauma team. Usually, a surgeon heads the team, and PAs perform duties such as collecting blood gases, putting in a chest tube, holding pressure on an arterial bleeder, and helping insert a central line. Not all PAs who work in the ER are directly involved with the trauma team. In fact, many hospitals require additional training for PAs who want to work in the area.

Major medicine is an area in which patients in need of acute medical attention are treated. Usually heart attack victims and patients in acute respiratory distress or cardiac arrest are triaged to the major medicine area. The PA may be the initial provider on the scene and will be responsible for initiating treatment until the attending physician arrives.

Fast track is an area designated for follow-up visits and routine, minor conditions like sore throats, coughs, hangnails, and so on. This is usually staffed by a designated PA on a daily basis or by several PAs who rotate through on different days.

The pediatric section of the ER is usually covered by the pediatric residents, interns, or PAs. The patients' ages range from newborn babies to teenagers. Common presentations include asthma attacks, sore throats, ear infections, and fevers. Obviously, the clinicians work closely with a patient's pediatrician to form a treatment plan. Usually, the surgical residents handle lacerations and broken bones.

Most ERs also have a psychiatric section for patients with acute psychiatric problems. That same area is often used for intoxicated patients or highly uncooperative or combative patients. The PA has a limited role in this area, except to contact the psychiatry department to have the patient evaluated. The PA may have to treat lacerations, bruises, or acute overdoses prior to the psychiatric evaluation.

The Team

The ER team consists of a variety of clinicians, technicians, nurses, clerical personnel, security, and personnel from various emergency medical services. The PAs work very closely with attending physicians, hospital staff, consulting physicians, nurses, and technicians to ensure the best treatment for the patient.

Salary

The PAs who work in the ER tend to be at the higher end of the pay scale, in part because of the stress of the job but also because of the number of hours and various shifts worked. The pay range is from $71,000 to $94,000 per year.

Summary

The ER PA must be able to work in a stressful environment in collaboration with a variety of team members. The job is fast paced and calls for clinicians who have both excellent surgical skills and thorough medical knowledge. Although there is usually a lot of backup available, given the high patient volume, many ER PAs work autonomously and require little supervision.

PEDIATRICS

Description of Duties

Pediatric PAs account for about 3% of the PA population, and work in clinics, private pediatrician offices, or in a hospital setting. In this section, we cover pediatric and neonatal PAs in the hospital setting, known as house staff.

For pediatric and neonatal PAs functioning as house staff, duties cover several areas and specialties. The PA is required to see patients on the in-patient pediatric floor, attend and assist with high-risk deliveries, evaluate and manage newborns (from 30 weeks' gestation onward), work in the pediatric clinic, and provide coverage to the ER as needed.

Usually, the job requires in-house calls and rotating shifts, as well as night and weekend shifts. As house staff, PAs may be the only clinicians available for emergencies in the middle of the night. Although the attending physician is always available by phone, the PA is often the first clinician on the scene to evaluate and stabilize the patient.

In pediatrics, patients are usually admitted through the ER or directly from a physician's office. The PA's duties on admission include performing a history and physical examination, ordering necessary tests, forming a diagnosis and treatment plan, and consulting with the attending pediatrician. The PA may also be required to draw blood samples, catheterize patients, and perform lumbar punctures. Daily follow-up with the patient, writing progress notes, and discussing further diagnostic and treatment modalities with the attending pediatrician are all parts of the PA's responsibilities.

In neonatology, the PA medically manages newborns from 30 weeks gestation until term. The supervising physician in this area is a neonatologist. Again, the PA's responsibility is to manage the day-to-day medical care of neonates, who have a variety of acute and chronic problems. This area is very procedure-oriented, with many intravenous starts, lumbar punctures, central (intravenous) line placements, ventilator management, collecting blood gases, placing chest tubes, and much more.

Attending high-risk deliveries is also a part of neonatology. Here, PAs are responsible for resuscitating newborns in the delivery room. Often, PAs work autonomously, with only the nursing staff available to revive infants until the anesthesiologist and pediatrician arrive.

The pediatric clinic is usually reserved for scheduled, nonemergency patients. This is where PAs perform well-baby checkups; give immunizations; and see a variety of colds, earaches, and sore throats. The acuteness of the patients is not as high as in neonatology, but the pace can be fast and furious.

Common calls to the emergency room are for asthma attacks, broken bones, and high fevers. On occasion, however, the PA may see a patient suffering from cardiac arrest or an acute overdose. In addition, many families without medical insurance bring their children to the emergency room for routine visits: colds, coughs, and rashes. Surgical injuries are usually deferred to surgical PAs or house staff.

The Team

The pediatric team consists of pediatricians, neonatologists, residents, interns, physician assistants, nurses, respiratory therapists, occupational therapists, nurse's aides, unit clerks, and secretaries.

Salary

Pediatric PAs tend to be at the middle of the pay scale with respect to PAs in other specialties. The range is from $64,000 to $87,000, depending on the hours worked.

Summary

The job of pediatric PA involves a lot of calm followed by moments of chaos. You must be willing and able to work various shifts, including nights, weekends, and holidays. The stress level ranges from extremely high when dealing with critically ill newborns to fairly routine when working in the clinic. You need to be well organized and, at times, ready to multitask. **This is not a job for PAs who lack confidence and maturity.**

PSYCHIATRY

Description of Duties

Psychiatry PAs generally work in either a hospital-based setting or in a clinic or mental health center. Approximately 3% of all PAs work in psychiatry.

In the hospital setting, PAs work in a consultation service or in the psychiatric ward of the facility. With consultation (consult) service, PAs evaluate inpatients from any area of the hospital—from surgery to medicine. Working closely with the psychiatrist in this setting, PAs evaluate patients for depression, anxiety, alcohol withdrawal, psychiatric medication problems, dementia, delirium, and, quite commonly with elderly intensive care patients, "sun downing." Many patients have a history of psychiatric illness and simply need to be followed while in the hospital. Others, however, may present new symptoms and require a more detailed work-up.

Once the PA evaluates a patient, the PA discusses the case with the attending or hospital-based psychiatrist and consults with the patient's attending physician as to the recommendation. Many times the recommendation is to change a medication or simply hold it for a period of time. Occasionally, the PA will recommend further testing, especially for patients who present with new findings. The PA may recommend a neurology consult or an MRI or CT scan to rule out certain pathology.

The PA will then follow all of the patients on the consult service, usually daily, writing notes and continuing recommendations until a patient is discharged or stable enough to not warrant further consultation.

The PAs working in the psychiatric ward of the hospital and a clinic or mental health center have similar duties and are covered together here. Many clinics treat a great deal of substance abuse (e.g., alcohol, drugs) patients and patients considered to have a dual diagnosis (e.g., substance abuse and psychiatric illness), for example, a patient suffering from alcoholism and schizophrenia. The patients may be treated on an inpatient or outpatient basis. The PA's role in this area is usually to take care of the patient's medical needs: physical examinations, monitoring of the patient's nonpsychiatric medications, hypertension, diabetes, seizures, and so on. The PA may also be responsible for teaching patients about topics such as AIDS, hepatitis, and nutrition.

Some PAs choose to work in this area because of the opportunity to be involved in research. Many clinics offer experimental drugs and/or treatment programs to patients who are struggling with alcohol or drug problems or who have not been successful with conventional treatment. The PA is more involved in counseling and group therapy than in the medical aspect of the treatment plan.

The Team

In a hospital setting (consult service), the PA works closely with the hospital psychiatrists, the patient's family, the nursing staff, and the patient's attending physician. In the clinic setting, the team consists of psychiatrists, psychologists, social workers, counselors, nurses, attending physicians (occasionally), technicians, and clerical personnel.

Salary

Psychiatry PAs tend to be at the mid-range of the pay scale. The average salary for a psychiatric PA is $76,948.

Summary

The psychiatric PA position is generally one of low stress. Hospital-based consult PAs work fairly autonomously, depending on their supervisor, and see a variety of patients throughout the hospital. The PA working in the psychiatric clinic usually works at a slow pace and can have a tedious job at times. This may be the perfect opportunity, however, for PAs interested in doing research and publishing papers.

OBSTETRICS AND GYNECOLOGY

Description of Duties

The ob-gyn specialty represents about 3% of the PA workforce. This specialty deals with both obstetrics (dealing with pregnant women during their pregnancy and childbirth) and gynecology (dealing with diseases peculiar to women, primarily those of the urinary tract as well as endocrinology and reproductive physiology). In this section, we discuss the role of the hospital-based ob-gyn PA.

This position is one of great diversity with respect to the various practice settings. The ob-gyn PA may work in a hospital's ob-gyn clinic, the operating room, the inpatient ob-gyn floor, the maternity ward, or sometimes in outreach (e.g., a community van that reaches out to the indigent population in the community).

In the ob-gyn clinic, the PA will see women for prenatal visits, annual Pap smears, pregnancy testing, and a variety of other complaints. The PA should be proficient in the pelvic examination. The ob-gyn PA should have excellent communication skills, particularly with teenagers, and the job requires a great deal of counseling with respect to teen pregnancy, HIV, and sexually transmitted diseases.

In the operating room, the PA is usually a first or second assistant to the attending ob-gyn physician. The majority of surgical cases include hysterectomies and laparoscopic explorations of the pelvic cavity. Also, PAs may have a role in assisting the attending physician in cesarean section deliveries.

The inpatient ob-gyn floor is generally reserved for patients recovering from surgery. The PA's role is to round on all of the patients, change dressings, check labs, write progress notes, and write orders. This function is very similar to that of the surgical PA.

The maternity ward is, of course, where most deliveries take place. In general, PAs have a limited role on this floor. The attending physician or midwife (who often plays a significant role in hospitals) deliver most babies.

Some hospitals and clinics do community outreach to provide routine and prenatal care to mothers who would not ordinarily come to a facility. This may be the only medical care many of these patients ever receive and is an excellent opportunity for PAs to make a difference in the community.

The Team

The ob-gyn field employs many more women than other specialties. In addition to PAs and MDs, the team may consist of nurse-practitioners, nurse midwives, nurses, technicians, operating room personnel, and clerical personnel.

Salary

Ob-gyn PAs tend to earn average salaries with respect to PAs in other areas. The range is from $53,000 to $84,000.

Summary

There is a great amount of diversity in ob-gyn, including surgery, medicine, inpatient, and clinic responsibilities. **The job can be both physically and mentally challenging, requiring both excellent diagnostic skills and proficient surgical capabilities.**

INTERNAL MEDICINE

Description of Duties

Approximately 8% of practicing PAs work in internal medicine. This section covers the hospital-based internal medicine PA. Keep in mind, though, that there are many opportunities available for PAs to work with private physicians and group practices.

The internal medicine PA must have, or acquire, a general understanding of all the medical subspecialties: cardiology, renal medicine, pulmonology, endocrinology, neurology, dermatology, hematology, and so on. As a result, **internal medicine is a great first job for new graduates who want to build a solid foundation for future practice.**

In the hospital environment, the internal medicine PA is usually a part of a team with other PAs and house staff (i.e., residents and interns). Next comes rounds with the chief resident.

The typical day starts early in the morning with individual rounds. Each clinician briefly sees and examines patients. Next comes rounds. The chief resident will gather the team and discuss each patient on the service. This usually takes place just outside of each patient's room. If a patient is new or has been admitted overnight, the primary provider will give a brief but thorough summary of the patient's history and physical examination, laboratory results, x-ray results, diagnosis, and treatment plan. The chief resident may then question the team or an individual member about issues relevant to the patient's case or presentation. This procedure is affectionately called "pimping," and it is a way to keep the entire team on its toes and makes for a great daily learning experience. Morning rounds can last from two to three hours, depending on the size of the service and the mood of the chief resident.

After team rounds, PAs generally have some time to check lab results and tests and to read notes in their patients' charts from consultants or the attending physician. The PAs then check any lab results or tests that may have been pending and begin to write the daily note on each patient. Included in the notes are the plan for the day and any specific orders that must be carried out as part of the treatment plan.

Throughout the day, the PA touches base with attending physicians and consulting physicians with respect to the patient's progress and treatment plan. The PA will also discuss any significant findings with the chief resident, who is ultimately responsible for the service.

At some point in the day, the team meets again for x-ray rounds. An attending radiologist usually presides over the meeting in the department of radiology and discusses each and every x-ray, ultrasound, MRI, angiogram, or CT scan performed on the patients on your service that morning. This is a great learning experience and helps the clinician get better acquainted with reading and interpreting various radiological studies.

In addition to team rounds and radiology rounds, the team may also have attending rounds. Usually, an attending physician is assigned to your service for the month and may give two or three lectures a week on various topics. This may include visiting with some patients and discussing their clinical findings. Again, this is an excellent and valuable learning tool.

Each PA is usually assigned one or two new admissions per day. For example, the PA goes to the ER and performs a complete history and physical exam on the patient. The PA then orders any appropriate tests (e.g., labs, x-rays), touches base with the attending physician, and writes the patient's admission orders. The patient is presented and discussed with the rest of the team at morning rounds.

In addition to the daily routine described previously, the internal medicine PA must also be proficient in various diagnostic and therapeutic procedures—obtaining blood gases, performing lumbar punctures, starting IVs, drawing blood, central line placement, and thoracentesis. Usually, the chief resident will teach these various procedures to PAs and allow them to accomplish them as proficiency and comfort level progress.

The Team

The internal medicine team consists of PAs, residents, interns, nurses, attending physicians, consulting physicians, technicians, aides, and clerical personnel.

Salary

The salary for internal medicine PAs tends to be in the mid range, usually because of the excellent hours and great teaching opportunities. The range is from $71,000 to $90,000.

Summary

This specialty offers great hours and low stress. In addition, it is a good job for new graduates because of the excellent learning opportunities available. Many PAs stay in the position for a couple of years and then move on to private practice or to a subspecialty due to the generalist nature of the position. This is definitely the perfect position for the cerebral PA.

SURGERY

Description of Duties

Surgery and its related subspecialties employ approximately 22% of PAs, second only to family practice. Physician assistants function effectively in multiple clinical settings, performing in-hospital surgical tasks along with and, not infrequently, in place of residents. **Many hospitals employ PAs as house officers in lieu of maintaining a surgical residency teaching program of MDs.**

Physician assistants who wish to pursue a career in surgery should be proficient in medicine. In a typical hospital surgical service, PAs, as house officers, are responsible for the pre-, intra-, and postoperative care of surgical patients. A given patient's preoperative state of health clearly will affect his or her intra- and postoperative care, as well as the overall prognosis. Timely identification of any preexisting conditions (e.g., diabetes mellitus, pulmonary disease, coronary artery disease, peripheral vascular disease, renal disease, liver disease, a compromised immune system), together with appropriate preoperative intervention, are critical to a favorable outcome. Similarly, there are myriad postoperative conditions that can arise: fever, pulmonary embolus, respiratory distress, renal failure, infection, and hemorrhage. These conditions can be lessened, or prevented, by the intervention of a knowledgeable surgical PA.

The responsibilities of the surgical PA include taking the patient's history, performing the physical exam, ordering appropriate tests and x-rays, writing admission orders, and performing a preoperative check prior to the patient's surgery. In addition, postoperatively, the PA does rounds on the floor, writes notes on all of the patients, changes the treatment plan as needed, and consults with the attending physician (surgeon) on a daily basis.

Intraoperatively, the PA's duties include first and second assisting. Many surgical procedures consist of the attending surgeon and the PA doing the actual surgery, with the ancillary help of the scrub nurse, circulating nurse, technicians, and anesthesiologist. **The surgical PA should have a thorough knowledge of anatomy and be technically proficient in various procedures.**

In addition to assisting with major surgical procedures, the surgical PA should be able to perform a variety of minor surgical and invasive procedures. These include but are not limited to administration of local anesthesia, surgical debridement of wounds, intramuscular injections and arthrocentesis, peripheral and central venous cannulation, chest tube placement and removal, proper immobilization of various fractured bones (and traction where indicated), bladder catheterization, and airway management and intubation. The surgical PA should also be able to perform and interpret electrocardiograms and be adult cardiac life support (ACLS) qualified.

The surgical PA is often called to the ER to evaluate and admit patients to the surgical service. The ability of the surgical PA to work in collaboration with the ER team is essential. Decisions made by the PA affect not only the patient's health but also the efforts of the nurses, lab technicians, respiratory therapists, physical and occupational therapists, and team members from other services in the hospital.

The surgical PA is usually required to take call on a rotating basis. This usually involves spending the night in the hospital, mostly in the surgical intensive care unit, and providing care to the entire service as needed.

The Team

The surgical team consists of a variety of medical and surgical personnel. Mostly, surgical PAs work with attending surgeons, nurses, various technicians and therapists, circulating nurses, scrub nurses, and anesthesiologists (or nurse anesthetists) in the operating room, along with medical attending physicians and various interns and residents.

Salary

Surgery PAs are usually on the higher end of the pay scale. This is usually because of the acuteness of the patients, the on-call hours, and the fact that attending physicians can be reimbursed for first assistant services. The range is from $69,000 to $93,000.

Summary

Being a surgical PA is definitely not a job for the shy and retiring. Surgical PAs are generally type A individuals. In addition, they must have excellent written and verbal communication skills, a willingness to handle responsibility, and the ability to be a team player. They must also be able to pay strict attention to detail.

What If I Don't Get In?

GRIEVING

Those of you who have taken classes in death and dying will be familiar with the five steps involved in the grieving process: denial, anger, bargaining, depression, and acceptance. Although being rejected from PA school does not compare with losing a family member, or even with losing a pet, it can still be a devastating and discouraging experience. The trick is to move through the process and get to the acceptance phase as quickly as possible. This will allow you to begin working toward improving your application for next year.

At first, you might have a hard time believing that after all of the hard work you put into the process, you weren't accepted. You may then become angry, realizing that your best-laid plans have been shattered. Your attitude may become self-defeating. The key here is not to burn any bridges, and by no means should you call the program and try to bargain or beg for acceptance. This will only hurt your chances for the next year. Believe me, there will be a next year, and it will come sooner than you think.

You will naturally be disappointed, but the sun will still rise tomorrow. Don't take things too personally—many excellent candidates don't get into PA school on their first try. It's mostly a matter of logistics: too many good applicants for precious few slots. Get through the grieving process and get ready to go back to work.

GATHER YOUR THOUGHTS

As I have tried to point out all through this book, only 5% of applicants are accepted each year. Is it the top 5% who get in? Hardly. No system is perfect, and some less qualified applicants are likely to slip through the cracks and be accepted. Many of these people will also fail along the way. This is inevitable, but some schools have a higher attrition rate than others. Take comfort in knowing that you're not alone and that you will get another chance.

In any case, keep a positive attitude. You will be a much stronger, and wiser, candidate next year. You will improve your grades, gain more experience, have a better understanding of the profession, and have more time to write a great essay.

DEVELOP A PLAN

Once you become ready to pick yourself up by the bootstraps, contact the schools that you applied to and ask for feedback on your application. This is a critical step, as you need to find out specifically the areas in which you are lacking as a candidate. Admissions committee members usually write down notes about your application or interview. Ask for specific areas that you need to improve on. Generally, the comments will be relevant to experience, grades, understanding of the profession, poor essay, poor interview, or behavior. The last may be hard to elicit from the program director or whoever gives you feedback. Make a note of any suggestions and thank the committee for considering your application or for the interview. It is important to do this right away while the application is still fresh in their minds.

Once you accomplish the above, you are ready to return to Chapter 3 and rewrite your goals. I hope by now you realize the value of doing this. Compile a concise plan of action to strengthen your application for next year. Do you need to take any classes over? Do you need more hands-on experience? How about your narrative—is it persuasive and motivating? Think carefully about how you can present yourself in a better light next year.

IMPLEMENT THE PLAN

Just do it! After you have a complete list of goals, begin working on them in the order of importance. For instance, if the program director told you that the committee was concerned with your ability to handle a rigorous science course load, enroll in some hard science classes. If you are lacking experience, go out and start volunteering in the local ER. As a volunteer, you are usually considered an insider by the hospital, and you may have a good shot at a paid job if one arises. Better yet, take a short course to become a certified nursing assistant and get a paid job in a hospital or clinic. Jobs usually abound in this field.

Remember, the committee will look to see what you have done to improve your application over the past year. Too many people apply over and over again but fail to make any positive changes.

NARRATIVE STATEMENT

When you fill out your application next year, be sure to write a new narrative statement and obtain fresh letters of recommendation. This is very important. Let the committee know exactly what you have done to improve and strengthen your application. Point out where you have followed their advice or taken an extra class or gained more hands-on experience.

Writing an Effective Letter of Recommendation

The purpose of a letter of recommendation is to provide the admissions committee with a detailed description of an applicant's abilities rather than merely checking off a few boxes on a standard form. Too many applicants feel that as long as the letter is written by a big shot, the content is irrelevant. This is simply not true, and a poorly composed letter may hinder rather than help your application.

Let's look at a sample letter of recommendation for a candidate applying to PA school. Afterward, we will dissect it and point out the three key elements that make up a great letter of reference.

> Dear Ms. Dean:
>
> Please accept this letter as a strong recommendation for John Smith's application as a student in your physician assistant program. I am the current dean of the College of Health and Human Performance at Mankato State University, and John was my student for four years and my teaching assistant for two years.
>
> As a student, John was easily in the top 10% of his peers for four years in a row. As a teaching assistant, he was rated highest by more than 122 students who have taken my classes. All students respected him and admired his presentations and leadership. He proved himself a dedicated, hardworking, and diligent young man.
>
> John served for four years in the U.S. Navy as a corpsman, and his experience in that position would give great strength to his career as a physician

assistant. He also spent time as an officer in the U.S. Air Force, which explains his admirable ability to pay strict attention to detail.

This young man has a social conscience, high energy, a cooperative style, and the uncanny ability to analyze complex problems in the health field in simple yet constructive context. His social graces are beyond reproach. John would make an outstanding PA. He really cares for people, and people care for him.

I strongly recommend John Smith for your physician assistant program.

Sincerely,

Robert R. Rockingham, Ph.D.
Dean, College of Health and Human Performance
Mankato State University

CONTENT

This letter contains the three key elements of an appropriate letter of reference:

1. Introduction and background of the writer
2. Writer's relationship to the candidate
3. Quantified claims rather than general statements

The purpose of the writer introducing him- or herself in the opening paragraph is to qualify as a legitimate reference. It shows that the reference truly knows the applicant and can honestly and objectively comment on the applicant's achievements, interpersonal and organizational skills, compassion, and so on.

Finally, the reference quantifies the applicant's claims. Many people make it seem like they can walk on water in their applications. If the writer uses "meaningful specifics" versus "wandering generalities," he or she lends more credence to the letter (e.g., "was rated the highest by more than 122 students".

IDENTIFY CANDIDATE'S STRENGTHS

A good recommendation letter does not simply recite the obvious: "Sue has a great GPA." It's quite obvious to the committee that Sue has a 3.7 GPA; they have her transcripts.

The writer should be more creative and spend enough time on the letter to make you stand out from the crowd. The writer is usually asked to evaluate you in several areas:

1. Academic performance
2. Interpersonal skills
3. Maturity
4. Adaptability and flexibility
5. Motivation for career as a PA

The writer may comment on all of those areas or just a couple. In the area that the writer does comment on, however, the statements should be specific and relevant to the category selected. For instance:

Academic performance: "top 10% of his peers."

Interpersonal skills: "He cares for people, and people care for him."

Maturity: "All students respected him and admired his presentations and leadership."

Adaptability and flexibility: "the uncanny ability to analyze complex problems . . . in simple yet constructive terms."

WHAT ABOUT WEAKNESSES?

Everyone has faults; the trick here is to have the evaluator mention a minor weakness and present it as though it were a strength. Mentioning a weakness lends objectivity and credibility to the letter of recommendation. Example: "John's strict attention to detail, at times, appeared to keep him late in the office. However, it is for this very reason that I believe he will make an excellent clinician and will not miss any details when it comes to taking care of his patients."

ONE FINAL TIP

The writer should keep in mind that the reader of your application may have to read a hundred others before yours. It's very important to keep the letters short, concise, specific, and personal. Be sure that the writer is recommending you for PA school and not medical school. Also, be sure that the writer changes the name of the school with each application you send in.

Personalized Goal Sheet

Fill out the following sheet and keep a copy with you at all times. Read this sheet every morning when you arise and every evening before you retire. By reviewing your goals daily, your subconscious mind will automatically begin working on helping you achieve them. This is a powerful technique, and it works!

My goal is to apply to the _____ PA program(s) and be accepted by _____. (Call each program that you will apply to and find out when candidates are notified about acceptance.)

To achieve this goal, I will have to overcome the following obstacles: **(List all of the obstacles that you are likely to encounter, such as financial, relocation, convincing a spouse/partner)**

_____

_____

_____

_____

The following people and organizations will help me achieve this goal: **(List everyone who can help you along the way: other PAs, the AAPA, your state chapter of the AAPA, friends, relatives, yourself)**

_____

_____

_____

To be a competitive candidate I will have to: (**What will it take for you to stand out from the crowd? For example, will you have to take more science courses, gain more experience, work on getting a great letter of reference?**)

_____

_____

_____

Beginning tonight, I will start putting into action the following plan: (**What can you do right now to get started?**)

_____

_____

_____

The benefits I will receive from achieving the goal of getting into the PA school of my choice include: (**Ask yourself, "What's in it for me? Why do I want to pursue this goal in the first place?"**)

_____

_____

_____

APPENDIX D

List of Synonyms

The following is a list of synonyms that will help you add more life and power to your essays. I encourage you to purchase a thesaurus and refer to it frequently or use the thesaurus in your word-processing program for help with language.

articulate: crystal clear, distinct, intelligible, eloquent, fluent, coherent

commitment: vow, assurance, obligation, guarantee, determination, promise

crusader: fighter, visionary, advocate, champion, zealot

dependable: reliable, trustworthy, faithful, steady

enthusiastic: intense, glowing, passionate, emotional

flexible: adaptable, conformable, adjustable, fluid, open-minded

integrity: honesty, veracity, candidness, honor

logical: rational, reasonable, consistent, valid

mature: refined, polished, self-sufficient, responsible, dependable, prudent

perceptive: sensitive, responsive, open, discriminating, insightful, quick, keen

poised: composed, calm, cool, well mannered, polished, suave, unflappable

practical: wise, tough, judicious, prudent, shrewd, canny, sharp, astute, clever

realistic: practical, pragmatic, commonsense, down-to-earth, sensible, rational

sincere: open, straight, earnest, fervent, dedicated, resolute, unpretentious

tactful: diplomatic, prudent, discreet, sensitive, clever, skillful, polished

teamwork: collaboration, interaction, cooperation, synergy, harmony, concert

APPENDIX E

AAPA State Constituent Chapters

Society of Air Force Physician Assistants
http://www.safpa.org/

Alabama Society of Physician Assistants
http://www.myaspa.org/

Alaska Academy of Physician Assistants
http://www.akapa.org/

Arizona State Association of Physician Assistants
http://www.asapa.org/

Arkansas Academy of Physician Assistants
http://www.arkansaspa.org/

Society of Army Physician Assistants
http://www.sapa.org/

California Academy of Physician Assistants
http://www.capanet.org/

Colorado Academy of Physician Assistants
http://www.coloradopas.org/

Connecticut Academy of Physician Assistants
http://www.connapa.org/

Delaware Academy of Physician Assistants
http://www.delawarepas.org/sbnctest2/

District of Columbia Academy of Physician Assistants
http://www.dcapa.org/

Florida Academy of Physician Assistants
http://www.fapaonline.org/

Georgia Association of Physician Assistants
http://www.gapa.net/

Hawaii Academy of Physician Assistants
http://www.hapahawaii.org/

Idaho Academy of Physician Assistants
http://www.idahopa.org/

Illinois Academy of Physician Assistants
http://www.illinoispa.org/

Indiana Academy of Physician Assistants
http://www.indianapas.org/

Iowa Physician Assistant Society
http://www.iapasociety.org/

Kansas Academy of Physician Assistants
http://www.kansaspa.com/

Kentucky Academy of Physician Assistants
http://www.kentuckypa.org/

Louisiana Academy of Physician Assistants
http://www.ourlapa.org/

Downeast Association of PAs
http://www.deapa.com/

Maryland Academy of Physician Assistants
http://www.mdapa.org/menumain.asp

Massachusetts Association of Physician Assistants
http://www.mass-pa.com/

Michigan Academy of Physician Assistants
http://www.michiganpa.org/AM/Template.cfm?Section=Home2

Minnesota Academy of Physician Assistants
http://www.mnacadpa.org/

Mississippi Academy of Physician Assistants
http://www.missipas.org/

Missouri Academy of Physician Assistants
http://www.moapa.org/

Montana Academy of Physician Assistants
http://www.mtapa.com/

Naval Association of Physician Assistants
http://www.napasite.net/

Nebraska Academy of Physician Assistants
http://www.nebraskapa.org/

Nevada Academy of Physician Assistants
http://www.nevadapa.com/

New Hampshire Society of Physician Assistants
http://www.nh-spa.org/

New Jersey State Society of Physician Assistants
http://www.njsspa.org/

New Mexico Academy of Physician Assistants
http://www.nmapa.com/

New York State Society of Physician Assistants
http://www.nysspa.org/

North Carolina Academy of Physician Assistants
http://www.ncapa.org/

North Dakota Academy of Physician Assistants
http://www.ndapahome.org/

Ohio Association of Physician Assistants
http://www.ohiopa.com/

Oklahoma Academy of Physician Assistants
http://www.okpa.org/

Oregon Society of Physician Assistants
http://www.oregonpa.org/

Pennsylvania Society of PAs
http://www.pspa.net/index.html

Public Health Service Academy of Physician Assistants
http://phsapa.com

Rhode Island Academy of Physician Assistants
http://www.myriapa.org/

South Carolina Academy of Physician Assistants
http://www.scapapartners.org/

South Dakota Academy of Physician Assistants
http://www.sdapa.net/

Tennessee Academy of Physician Assistants
http://www.tnpa.com/

Texas Academy of Physician Assistants
http://www.tapa.org/

Utah Academy of Physician Assistants
http://www.utahapa.org/

Physician Assistant Academy of Vermont
http://www.paav.org/

Veterans Affairs Physician Assistant Association
http://www.vapaa.org/

Virginia Academy of Physician Assistants
http://www.vapa.org/

Washington State Academy of Physician Assistants
http://www.wapa.com/

West Virginia Association of Physician Assistants
http://www.mywvapa.org/

Wisconsin Academy of Physician Assistants
http://www.wapa.org/

Wyoming Association of Physician Assistants
http://www.wapa.net/

APPENDIX F

U.S. PA Programs Accredited by ARC-PA

This information provided by the ARC-PA at http://www.arc-pa.com/acc_programs/index.html.

ALABAMA

University of Alabama at Birmingham
Surgical Physician Assistant Program
School of Health Related Professions
RMSB 481; 1530 3rd Avenue South
Birmingham, AL
35294-1212
Phone: (205) 934-4605
http://main.uab.edu/Shrp/Default.aspx?pid=32650

University of South Alabama
Department of Physician Assistant Studies
1504 Springhill Avenue, Suite 4410
Mobile, AL
36604-3273
Phone: (251) 434-3641
http://www.southalabama.edu/alliedhealth/pa/

ARIZONA

Arizona School of Health Sciences
Physician Assistant Program
5850 East Still Circle
Mesa, AZ
85206
Phone: (480) 219-6000

http://www.atsu.edu/ashs/programs/physician_assistant/napa.htm

Midwestern University
Office of Admissions
Physician Assistant Program
19555 North 59th Avenue
Glendale, AZ
85308-6813

http://www.midwestern.edu/Programs_and_Admission/
AZ_Physician_Assistant_Studies.html

ARKANSAS

Harding University
Physician Assistant Program
Box 12231
Searcy, AR
72149
Phone: (501) 279-5642

http://www.harding.edu/PAprogram/

ARMED FORCES

Interservice Physician Assistant Program
Academy of Health Sciences
Attn: MCCSHMP
3151 Scott Road, Suite 1302
Fort Sam Houston, TX, UN
78234-6138
Phone: (210) 221-8004

http://www.usarec.army.mil/armypa/

CALIFORNIA

Charles R. Drew University of Medicine and Science
Physician Assistant Program
College of Health Sciences
1731 East 120th Street
Los Angeles, CA
90059
Phone: (323) 563-5879

http://www.allalliedhealthschools.com/find/show.php?id=1672

Keck School of Medicine of the University of Southern California
Physician Assistant Program
Department of Family Medicine
1000 South Fremont Avenue, Unit 7, Bldg. A-6, Rm. 6429
Alhambra, CA
91803-8897
Phone: (626) 457-4240

http://www.usc.edu/schools/medicine/departments/ physician_assistant/

Loma Linda University
Physician Assistant Program
School of Allied Health Professions
Nichol Hall, Room 2033
Loma Linda, CA
92350
Phone: (909) 558-7295

http://www.llu.edu/llu/sahp/pa/

Riverside County Regional Medical Center/Riverside Community College
Primary Care PA Program
16130 Lasselle Street
Moreno Valley, CA
92551
Phone: (951) 571-6166

http://www.rcc.edu/academicPrograms/physicianAssistant/

Samuel Merritt University
Physician Assistant Program
450 30th Street, Ste. 4708
Oakland, CA
94609
Phone: (510) 869-6623

http://www.samuelmerritt.edu/physician_assistant

San Joaquin Valley College
Primary Care PA Program
8400 West Mineral King Avenue
Visalia, CA
93291
Phone: (559) 651-2500 ext. 351

http://www.sjvc.edu/programs/programs.php?programID=26

Stanford University School of Medicine
Primary Care Associate Program
Family Nurse Practitioner
Physician Assistant Program
1215 Welch Road, Modular G
Palo Alto, CA
94305-5408
Phone: (650) 725-6959

http://pcap.stanford.edu/program/pa.html

Touro University—California College of Health Sciences
Physician Assistant Program
Office of Admissions
1310 Johnson Lane
Vallejo, CA
94592
Phone: (888) 652-7580

http://www.tu.edu/departments.php?id=50&page=610

University of California—Davis
Physician Assistant Program
Family Nurse Practitioner Program
Department of Family and Community Medicine
2516 Stockton Blvd, Suite 254
Sacramento, CA
95817-2208
Phone: (916) 734-3551

http://www.ucdmc.ucdavis.edu/fnppa/

Western University of Health Sciences
Primary Care Physician Assistant Program
309 E. Second Street
Pomona, CA
91766-1854
Phone: (909) 469-5378

http://www.westernu.edu/xp/edu/cahp/mspas_about.xml

COLORADO

Red Rocks Community College
Physician Assistant Program
13300 West 6th Avenue
Denver, CO
80228-1255
Phone: (303) 914-6386

http://www.rrcc.edu/pa/

University of Colorado at Denver and Health Sciences Center
Child Health Associate
Physician Assistant Program
PO Box 6508, Mail Stop F543
Aurora, CO
80045
Phone: (303) 315-7963

http://www.uchsc.edu/chapa/

CONNECTICUT

Quinnipiac University
Physician Assistant Program
Office of Graduate Admissions (AB-GRD)
275 Mount Carmel Avenue
Hamden, CT
06518-1908
Phone: (203) 582-8672

http://www.quinnipiac.edu/x781.xml

Yale University School of Medicine
Physician Associate Program
367 Cedar Street
Harkness Office Building, 2nd Floor
New Haven, CT
06510
Phone: (203) 785-2860

http://medicine.yale.edu/pa/

WASHINGTON, D.C.

George Washington University
Physician Assistant Program
900 23rd Street NW, Suite 6148
Washington, DC
20037
Phone: (202) 994-6661

http://www.gwumc.edu/healthsci/programs/pa/

Howard University
Physician Assistant Program
College of Pharmacy, Nursing and Allied Health Sciences
6th & Bryant Street, NW, Annex I
Washington, DC
20059
Phone: (202) 806-7536

http://www.cpnahs.howard.edu/AHS/Pa/Introduction.htm

FLORIDA

Barry University School of Graduate Medical Sciences
Physician Assistant Program
11300 NE Second Avenue, Box SGMS
Miami Shores, FL
33161
Phone: (305) 899-3296
http://www.barry.edu/pa/

Miami Dade College
Physician Assistant Program
Medical Center Campus
950 NW 20th Street
Miami, FL
33127-4693
Phone: (305) 237-4124
http://www.mdc.edu/medical/academic_programs/physician_assistant/physician.htm

Nova Southeastern University, Ft. Lauderdale
Physician Assistant Program
3200 South University Dr.
Fort Lauderdale, FL
33328
Phone: (954) 262-1250
http://www.nova.edu/pa/

Nova Southeastern University, Jacksonville
Physician Assistant Program
6675 Corporate Center Parkway, Suite 112
Jacksonville, FL
32216
Phone: (904) 245-8990
http://www.nova.edu/pa/jacksonville/

Nova Southeastern University, Orlando
Physician Assistant Program
4850 Millenia Boulevard
Orlando, FL
32839
Phone: (407) 264-5150
http://www.nova.edu/pa/orlando/

Nova Southeastern University, Southwest Florida
Physician Assistant Program
2655 Northbrooke Drive
Naples, FL
34119
Phone: (239) 591-4528 ext. 20
http://www.nova.edu/pa/swflorida/

University of Florida
Physician Assistant Program
PO Box 100176
Gainesville, FL
32610-0176
Phone: (352) 265-7955
http://www.med.ufl.edu/pap/apply/

GEORGIA
Emory University School of Medicine
Physician Assistant Program
Department of Family and Preventive Medicine
1462 Clifton Rd, Suite 280
Atlanta, GA
30322
Phone: (404) 727-7825
http://www.emorypa.org/

Medical College of Georgia
Physician Assistant Program
Physician Assistant Department
EC-3304
Augusta, GA
30912
Phone: (706) 721-3246
http://www.mcg.edu/students/semcon/corefpa.htm

Mercer University College of Pharmacy and Health Sciences
Physician Assistant Program
3001 Mercer University Drive
Atlanta, GA
30341
Phone: (678-547-6214
http://cophs.mercer.edu/pa.htm

South University
Physician Assistant Program
709 Mall Blvd.
Savannah, GA
31406
Phone: (912) 201-8025
http://www.southuniversity.edu/PhysicianAssistant/

IDAHO

Idaho State University
Department of Physician Assistant Studies
Campus Box 8253
1021 S Red Hill Road
Pocatello, ID
83209-8253
Phone: (208) 282-4726
http://www.isu.edu/PAprog/

IOWA

Des Moines University
Physician Assistant Program
3200 Grand Avenue
Des Moines, IA
50312
Phone: (515) 271-7854

http://www.dmu.edu/chs/pa/

University of Iowa
Physician Assistant Program
Carver College of Medicine
5167 Westlawn
Iowa City, IA
52242-1100
Phone: (319) 335-8922

http://paprogram.medicine.uiowa.edu/

ILLINOIS

**John H. Stroger Jr. Hospital of Cook County/
Malcolm X College**
Physician Assistant Program
1900 W. Van Buren, #3241
Chicago, IL
60612
Phone: (312) 850-7255

**http://malcolmx.ccc.edu/Academic_Programs/
PhysicianAssistant.asp**

Midwestern University
Physician Assistant Program
555 31st Street
Downers Grove, IL
60515
Phone: (800) 458-6253

**http://www.midwestern.edu/Programs_and_Admission/
IL_Physician_Assistant_Studies.html**

Rosalind Franklin University of Medicine and Science
Physician Assistant Program
3333 Green Bay Road
North Chicago, IL
60064-3095
Phone: (847) 589-8686
**http://www.rosalindfranklin.edu/DNN/home/CHP/PA/MS/
tabid/1570/Default.aspx**

Southern Illinois University at Carbondale
Physician Assistant Program
Lindegren Hall, Room 129, Mail Code 6516
Carbondale, IL
62901-6516
Phone: (618) 453-5527
http://www.siu.edu/~sah/pa.html

INDIANA
Butler University/Clarian Health
Physician Assistant Program
College of Pharmacy and Health Sciences
4600 Sunset Avenue
Indianapolis, IN
46208
Phone: (317) 940-9969
http://www.butler.edu/cophs/?pg=2077&parentID=2041

University of Saint Francis
Physician Assistant Program
2701 Spring Street
Fort Wayne, IN
46808
Phone: (260) 434-7737
http://www.sf.edu/healthscience/pa/msentryprogram.shtml

KANSAS

Wichita State University
Physician Assistant Program
College of Health Professions
1845 N. Fairmount, Box 43
Wichita, KS
67260-0043
Phone: (316) 978-3011

http://webs.wichita.edu/?u=chp_pa&p=/index

KENTUCKY

University of Kentucky
Physician Assistant Program
College of Health Sciences
900 S. Limestone Street, Suite 205
Lexington, KY
40536-0200
Phone: (859) 323-1100

http://www.mc.uky.edu/PA/

LOUISIANA

Louisiana State University Health Sciences Center
Physician Assistant Program
School of Allied Health Professions
1501 Kings Highway, PO Box 33932
Shreveport, LA
71130-3932
Phone: (318) 675-7317

**http://www.universities.com/edu/Louisiana_State_University_
Health_Sciences_Center_Bachelor_degree_Physician_Assistant.html**

Our Lady of the Lake College
Physician Associate Program
7443 Picardy Avenue
Baton Rouge, LA
70808
Phone: (225) 214-6988

http://www.ololcollege.edu/physician_asst.html

MASSACHUSETTS

Massachusetts College of Pharmacy and Health Sciences
Physician Assistant Studies Program
179 Longwood Avenue, W110
Boston, MA
02115
Phone: (617) 732-2918

http://www.mcphs.edu/academics/programs/physician_assistant_studies/

Northeastern University
Physician Assistant Program
360 Huntington Ave
202 Robinson Hall
Boston, MA
02115
Phone: (617) 373-3195

http://www.northeastern.edu/bouve/programs/mphysassist/mphysassist.html

Springfield College/Baystate Health System
Physician Assistant Program
263 Alden Street
Springfield, MA
01109
Phone: (800) 343-1257

http://catalog.spfldcol.edu/preview_program.php?catoid=26&poid=891&bc=1

MARYLAND

Anne Arundel Community College
Physician Assistant Program
School of Health Professions, Wellness and Physical Education
101 College Parkway
Arnold, MD
21012
Phone: (410) 777-7310

http://www.aacc.edu/physassist/Admissions.cfm

Towson University, CCBC Essex
Physician Assistant Program
7201 Rossville Boulevard
Baltimore, MD
21237-1899
Phone: (410) 780-6159

http://www.towson.edu/chp/pa/

University of Maryland, Eastern Shore
Physician Assistant Program
Haze Hall, Room 1034
Princess Anne, MD
21853
Phone: (410) 651-7584

http://www.umes.edu/PA/Default.aspx?id=2408

MAINE

University of New England
Physician Assistant Program
716 Stevens Avenue
Biddeford, ME
04103-7688
Phone: (207) 221-4529

http://www.une.edu/chp/pa/

MICHIGAN

Central Michigan University
Physician Assistant Program
1222 Health Professions Bldg
Mount Pleasant, MI
48859
Phone: (989) 774-2478

**http://www.gradschools.com/Program/MI_United-States/
Graduate-Program-Physician-Assistant/205187.html**

Grand Valley State University
Physician Assistant Program
301 Michigan Street, NE, Ste. 200 CHS
Grand Rapids, MI
49503
Phone: (616) 331-3356
http://www.gvsu.edu/pas/

University of Detroit Mercy
Physician Assistant Program
4001 West McNichols Road
Detroit, MI
48221
Phone: (313) 993-2474
http://www.udmercy.edu/apply/financial_aid/type/
health-professions/physician-assistant/index.htm

Wayne State University
Department of Physician Assistant Studies
259 Mack Avenue, Ste. 2590
Detroit, MI
48201
Phone: (313) 577-1368
http://www.pa.cphs.wayne.edu/

Western Michigan University
Physician Assistant Program
1903 West Michigan Avenue
Kalamazoo, MI
49008-5138
Phone: (269) 387-5314
http://www.wmich.edu/paprog/

MINNESOTA

Augsburg College
Physician Assistant Program
Campus Box 149
2211 Riverside Avenue
Minneapolis, MN
55454
Phone: (612) 330-1399

http://www.augsburg.edu/pa/

MISSOURI

Missouri State University
Department of Physician Assistant Studies
901 S. National PTPA 112
Springfield, MO
65897
Phone: (417) 836-6151

http://www.missouristate.edu/pas/

Saint Louis University
Physician Assistant Program
Doisy College of Health Sciences
3437 Caroline Street
St. Louis, MO
63104-1111
Phone: (314) 977-8521

http://www.slu.edu/x2348.xml

MONTANA

Rocky Mountain College
Physician Assistant Program
1511 Poly Drive
Billings, MT
59102-1739
Phone: (406) 657-1190

http://www.rocky.edu/academics/programs/mpas/Admissions.shtml

NORTH CAROLINA

Duke University Medical Center
Physician Assistant Program
DUMC 3848
Durham, NC
27710
Phone: (919) 681-3161

http://paprogram.mc.duke.edu/

East Carolina University
Physician Assistant Program
School of Allied Health Sciences
Health Sciences Building, Suite 4310
Greenville, NC
27858-4353
Phone: (252) 744-1100

http://www.ecu.edu/pa/

Methodist University
Physician Assistant Program
5107B College Centre Drive
Fayetteville, NC
28311
Phone: (910) 630-7495

http://www.methodist.edu/paprogram/

Wake Forest University
Physician Assistant Program
Medical Center Boulevard
Winston-Salem, NC
27157-1006
Phone: (336) 716-4356

http://www1.wfubmc.edu/PAprogram/

Wingate University
Physician Assistant Program
Campus Box 5010
Wingate, NC
28174
Phone: (704) 233-8051
http://pa.wingate.edu/

NORTH DAKOTA

University of North Dakota School of Medicine and Health Sciences
Physician Assistant Program
Department of Family and Community Medicine
501 N. Columbia Road—Stop 9037, Room 4128
Grand Forks, ND
58202-9037
Phone: (701) 777-2344
http://www.med.und.nodak.edu/physicianassistant/

NEBRASKA

Union College
Physician Assistant Program
3800 South 48th Street
Lincoln, NE
68506
Phone: (402) 486-2527
http://www.ucollege.edu/?DivID=1&pgID=301

University of Nebraska Medical Center
Physician Assistant Program
984300 Nebraska Medical Center
Omaha, NE
68198-4300
Phone: (402) 559-9495
http://www.unmc.edu/alliedhealth/pa/

NEW HAMPSHIRE

Massachusetts College of Pharmacy and Health Sciences, Manchester
PA Program
1260 Elm Street
Manchester, NH
03101
Phone: (603) 314-1730

http://www.mcphs.edu/academics/programs/ physician_assistant_studies/PA_24_Man/

NEW JERSEY

Seton Hall University
Physician Assistant Program
400 South Orange Avenue
South Orange, NJ
07079-2689
Phone: (973) 275-2596

http://www.shu.edu/academics/gradmeded/ ms-physician-assistant/index.cfm

University of Medicine and Dentistry of New Jersey
Physician Assistant Program
Robert Wood Johnson Medical School
675 Hoes Lane
Piscataway, NJ
08854-5635
Phone: (732) 235-4445

http://shrp.umdnj.edu/programs/paweb/

NEW MEXICO

University of New Mexico School of Medicine
Physician Assistant Program
Family & Community Medicine
MSC 09 5040, 1 University of New Mexico
Albuquerque, NM
87131-0001
Phone: (505) 272-9678
http://hsc.unm.edu/SOM/fcm/pap/

University of St. Francis
Physician Assistant Program
4401 Silver Avenue, SE, Suite B
Albuquerque, NM
87108
Phone: (888) 446-4657
http://www1.stfrancis.edu/content/conah/pa/

NEVADA

Touro University, Nevada
Physician Assistant Program
College of Osteopathic Medicine
874 American Pacific Drive
Henderson, NV
89014
Phone: (702) 777-1770
http://en.wikipedia.org/wiki/Physician_Assistant

NEW YORK

Albany Medical College
Physician Assistant Program
Center for Physician Assistant Studies
47 New Scotland Avenue, Mail Code 4
Albany, NY
12208-3412
Phone: (518) 262-5251
http://www.amc.edu/Academic/PhysicianAssistant/index.html

CUNY York College
Physician Assistant Program
94-20 Guy Brewer Blvd, Room 112 SC
Jamaica, NY
11451
Phone: (718) 262-2823

**http://york.cuny.edu/academics/departments/health-professions/
program-courses/physician-assistant-program**

D'Youville College
Physician Assistant Program
320 Porter Avenue
Buffalo, NY
14201
Phone: (716) 829-7713

http://www.dyc.edu/academics/physician_assistant/index.asp

Daemen College
Physician Assistant Department
4380 Main Street
Amherst, NY
14226-3592
Phone: (800) 462-7652

http://www.daemen.edu/academics/physician_assistant/

Hofstra University
Physician Assistant Studies Program
113 Monroe Lecture Hall
127 Hofstra University
Hempstead, NY
11549
Phone: (516) 463-4074

http://www.hofstra.edu/Academics/Colleges/HCLAS/PAP/

Le Moyne College
Physician Assistant Program
Department of Biology
1419 Salt Springs Road
Syracuse, NY
13214-1399
Phone: (315) 445-4745

http://www.lemoyne.edu/tabid/654/Default.aspx

Long Island University
Physician Assistant Program
121 DeKalb Avenue
Brooklyn, NY
11201
Phone: (718) 260-2780

http://www.brooklyn.liu.edu/health/bsphyass.html

Mercy College
Graduate Program in Physician Assistant Studies
1200 Waters Place
Bronx, NY
10461
Phone: (914) 674-7635

https://contest.mercy.edu/pages/865.asp

New York Institute of Technology
Physician Assistant Program
Riland Building, Suite 352—Northern Blvd
Old Westbury, NY
11568-8000
Phone: (516) 686-3881

http://www.nyit.edu/physician_assistant_studies/

Pace University-Lenox Hill Hospital
Physician Assistant Program
One Pace Plaza, Room Y-31
New York, NY
10038
Phone: (212) 346-1357

http://www.pace.edu/page.cfm?doc_id=6594

Rochester Institute of Technology
Physician Assistant Program
85 Lomb Memorial Drive
Rochester, NY
14623-5603
Phone: (584) 475-2978

http://www.rit.edu/cos/medical/physician_assistant.html

SUNY/Downstate Medical Center
Physician Assistant Program
Health Science Center
450 Clarkson Avenue—Box 1222
Brooklyn, NY
11203
Phone: (718) 270-2324) 5

http://www.downstate.edu/pa/

St. John's University
Physician Assistant Education Program
Dr. Andrew Bartilucci Center
175-05 Horace Harding Expressway
Fresh Meadows, NY
11365
Phone: (718) 990-8417

**http://www.stjohns.edu/admission/undergraduate/learnmore/
physassist**

Stony Brook University, SUNY
Physician Assistant Program
School of Health Technology & Management
SHTM—HSC, L2-424
Stony Brook, NY
11794-8202
Phone: (631) 444-3190 ext. 6

http://www.hsc.stonybrook.edu/shtm/pa/index.cfm

Sophie Davis School of Biomedical Education
CUNY Medical School
Harlem Hospital Center
138th Street and Convent Ave, Harris Hall, Suite G15
New York, NY
10031
Phone: (212) 650-7745

**http://www1.ccny.cuny.edu/prospective/med/programs/
paprogram.cfm**

Touro College
Physician Assistant Program
School of Health Sciences
1700 Union Blvd.
Bay Shore, NY
11706
Phone: (631) 665-1600

http://www.touro.edu/shs/pa.asp

Touro College, Manhattan Campus
Physician Assistant Program
School of Health Sciences
27-33 West 23rd Street
New York, NY
10010
Phone: (212) 463-0400, ext. 792

http://www.touro.edu/shs/pany/

Wagner College/Staten Island University Hospital
Physician Assistant Program
One Campus Road
Staten Island, NY
10301
Phone: (718) 420-4142 or 4151
http://www.wagner.edu/departments/pa_program/3yrPA

Weill Cornell Medical College
Physician Assistant Program (A Surgical Focus)
575 Lexington Avenue, Suite 600
New York, NY
10022
Phone: (646) 962-7277
http://www.med.cornell.edu/education/programs/phy_ass.html

OHIO

Cuyahoga Community College
Physician Assistant Program
11000 Pleasant Valley Road
Parma, OH
44130
Phone: (216) 987-5363
**http://www.tri-c.edu/programs/physicianassistant/Pages/
default.aspx**

Kettering College of Medical Arts
Physician Assistant Program
3737 Southern Boulevard
Kettering, OH
45429
Phone: (937) 296-7238
http://www.kcma.edu/academics/pa/index.html

Marietta College
Physician Assistant Program
215 Fifth Street
Marietta, OH
45750
Phone: (740) 376-4458
http://www.marietta.edu/~paprog/

Mount Union College
Physician Assistant Program
1972 Clark Avenue
Alliance, OH
44601
Phone: (800) 334-6682
**http://www2.muc.edu/Newsroom/February08/
physician_assistant_master_program_first_since_1912.aspx**

University of Findlay
Physician Assistant Program
1000 North Main Street
Findlay, OH
45840-3695
Phone: (419) 434-4529
**http://www.findlay.edu/academics/colleges/cohp/
academicprograms/undergraduate/PHAS/default.htm**

University of Toledo
Physician Assistant Program
School of Allied Health
3015 Arlington Avenue
Toledo, OH
43614-5803
Phone: (419) 383-5408
http://www.utoledo.edu/hshs/pa/index.html

OKLAHOMA

University of Oklahoma
Physician Assistant Program
Health Sciences Center
PO Box 26901
Oklahoma City, OK
73190
Phone: (405) 271-2058

http://www.okpa.org/Default.aspx?alias=www.okpa.org/paprogram

University of Oklahoma, Tulsa
Physician Assistant Program
4502 E. 41st Street
Tulsa, OK
74135-2512
Phone: (918) 619-4760

http://tulsa.ou.edu/pa/

OREGON

Oregon Health Sciences University
Physician Assistant Program
3181 SW Sam Jackson Park Road
GH219
Portland, OR
97239-3098
Phone: (503) 494-1484

**http://www.ohsu.edu/xd/education/schools/school-of-medicine/
academic-programs/physician-assistant/index.cfm**

Pacific University
Physician Assistant Program
School of Physician Assistant Studies
2043 College Way
Forest Grove, OR
97116
Phone: (503) 352-2898

http://www.pacificu.edu/pa/

PENNSYLVANIA

Arcadia University
Physician Assistant Program
Brubaker Hall, Health Science Center
450 South Easton Road
Glenside, PA
19038
Phone: (215) 572-2082

http://www.arcadia.edu/academic/default.aspx?id=425

Chatham College
Physician Assistant Program
Woodland Road
Pittsburgh, PA
15232
Phone: (412) 365-1412

http://www.chatham.edu/departments/healthmgmt/graduate/pa/

DeSales University
Physician Assistant Program
2755 Station Avenue
Center Valley, PA
18034-9568
Phone: (610) 282-1100 x1415

http://www.desales.edu/physician_assistant_studies_degree_pa.aspx

Drexel University Hahnemann
Physician Assistant Program
College of Nursing and Health Professions
1505 Race Street, 8th Floor, MS 504
Philadelphia, PA
19102-1192
Phone: (215) 762-7135

http://www.drexel.edu/cnhp/physician_assistant/masters_about.asp

Duquesne University
Physician Assistant Program
John G. Rangos, Sr., School of Health Sciences
323 Health Sciences Building
Pittsburgh, PA
15282

http://www.healthsciences.duq.edu/pa/pahome.html

Gannon University
Physician Assistant Program
109 University Square
Erie, PA
16541-0001
Phone: (814) 871-7474

http://www.gannon.edu/PROGRAMS/UNDER/phyasst.asp

King's College
Physician Assistant Program
133 North River Street
Wilkes-Barre, PA
18711
Phone: (570) 208-5853

www.kings.edu/paprog

Lock Haven University of Pennsylvania
Physician Assistant Program
Lock Haven, PA
17745
Phone: (570) 893-2541

http://gradprograms.lhup.edu/pa/

Marywood University
Physician Assistant Program
2300 Adams Avenue
Scranton, PA
18509
Phone: (570) 348-6298

http://www.marywood.edu/pa-program/

Pennsylvania College of Optometry
Physician Assistant Program
8360 Old York Road
Elkins Park, PA
19027
Phone: (215) 780-1515
http://www.salus.edu/images/pa/health_science.html

Pennsylvania College of Technology
Physician Assistant Program
DIF #123
One College Avenue
Williamsport, PA
17701-5799
Phone: (570) 327-4779
http://www.pct.edu/

Philadelphia College of Osteopathic Medicine
Department of Physician Assistant Studies
4190 City Avenue, Rowland Hall
Philadelphia, PA
19131
Phone: (215) 871-6772
**http://www.pcom.edu/academic_programs/aca_pa/degree_
programs_physician_assi/degree_programs_physician_assi.html**

Philadelphia University
Physician Assistant Program
School House Lane & Henry Avenue
Philadelphia, PA
19144
Phone: (215) 951-2908
http://www.philau.edu/PAProgram/

Saint Francis University
Department of Physician Assistant Sciences
PO Box 600
Loretto, PA
15940-0600
Phone: (814) 472-3020
http://www.francis.edu/MPAShome.htm

Seton Hill University
Physician Assistant Program
Seton Hill Drive
Greensburg, PA
15601
Phone: (724) 838-4283
http://www.setonhill.edu/academics/pa/index.cfm

SOUTH CAROLINA
Medical University of South Carolina
Physician Assistant Program
College of Health Professions
PO Box 250856
Charleston, SC
29425
Phone: (843) 792-1913
http://www.musc.edu/chp/pa/

SOUTH DAKOTA
University of South Dakota
Physician Assistant Studies Program
School of Medicine
414 East Clark Street
Vermillion, SD
57069-2390
Phone: (605) 677-5128
http://www.usd.edu/pa/

TENNESSEE

Bethel College
Physician Assistant Program
325 Cherry Avenue, Box 329
McKenzie, TN
38201
Phone: (731) 352-5708

http://www.bethel-college.edu/bethelpa/index.htm

Lincoln Memorial University—DeBusk College of Osteopathic Medicine
Physician Assistant Program
6965 Cumberland Gap Parkway
Harrogate, TN
37752

http://www.lmunet.edu/DCOM/pa/index.htm

South College
Master of Health Science—Physician Assistant Program
3904 Lonas Drive
Knoxville, TN
37909
Phone: (865) 251-1800

http://www.southcollegetn.edu/masters/physician-assistant/

Trevecca Nazarene University
Physician Assistant Program
333 Murfreesboro Road
Nashville, TN
37210-2877
Phone: (615) 248-1225

http://www.trevecca.edu/pa

TEXAS

Baylor College of Medicine
Physician Assistant Program
Room 107 BTXX, One Baylor Plaza
Houston, TX
77030-3498
Phone: (713) 798-4842
http://www.bcm.edu/pap/

Texas Tech University Health Sciences Center
School of Allied Health, Department of Diagnostic & Primary Care
Physician Assistant Program
3600 North Garfield
Midland, TX
79705
Phone: (915) 620-9905
http://www.ttuhsc.edu/sah/mpa/

University of Texas, Pan American
Physician Assistant Studies Program
1201 W. University Drive
Edinburg, TX
78539
Phone: (956) 381-2298
http://portal.utpa.edu/utpa_main/daa_home/hshs_home/pasp_home

University of Texas Health Science Center at San Antonio
Physician Assistant Program
Department of Physician Assistant Studies
7703 Floyd Curl Drive, MC 6249
San Antonio, TX
78229-3900
Phone: (210) 567-8811
http://www.uthscsa.edu/shp/pa/

University of Texas Medical Branch
Physician Assistant Program
School of Allied Health Services
301 University Boulevard
Galveston, TX
77555-1145
Phone: (409) 772-3046
http://www.sahs.utmb.edu/PAS/

University of North Texas
Physician Assistant Studies
Health Science Center at Fort Worth
3500 Camp Bowie Boulevard
Fort Worth, TX
76107-2699
Phone: (817) 735-2301
http://www.hsc.unt.edu/education/PASP/

University of Texas, Southwestern Medical Center at Dallas
Physician Assistant Program
6011 Harry Hines Boulevard
Dallas, TX
75390-9090
Phone: (214) 648-1701
http://www.utsouthwestern.edu/utsw/cda/dept48945/files/54102.html

UTAH
University of Utah
Physician Assistant Program
375 Chipeta Way
Salt Lake City, UT
84108
Phone: (801) 581-7766
http://web.utah.edu/upap/

VIRGINIA

Eastern Virginia Medical School
Physician Assistant Program
700 West Olney Road, Suite 1110
PO Box 1980
Norfolk, VA
23501-1980
Phone: (757) 446-7158

http://www.evms.edu/hlthprof/mpa/

James Madison University
Physician Assistant Program
Dept of Health Sciences, MSC 4301
Harrisonburg, VA
22807
Phone: (540) 568-2395

http://www.jmu.edu/healthsci/paweb/

Jefferson College of Health Sciences
Physician Assistant Program
920 S. Jefferson Street
Roanoke, VA
24016
Phone: (540) 985-4016

http://www.jchs.edu/page.php/prmID/77

Shenandoah University
Division of Physician Assistant Studies
1460 University Drive
Winchester, VA
22601
Phone: (540) 542-6208

http://www.su.edu/

WASHINGTON

University of Washington
MEDEX Northwest
Physician Assistant Program
4311 11th Ave NE, Suite 200
Seattle, WA
98105-4608
Phone: (206) 616-4001

http://www.washington.edu/medicine/som/depts/medex/

WISCONSIN

Marquette University
Department of Physician Assistant Studies
College of Health Sciences
1700 Building—PO Box 1881
Milwaukee, WI
53201-1881
Phone: (414) 288-5688

http://www.marquette.edu/chs/pa/index.shtml

University of Wisconsin, LaCrosse; Gunderson Lutheran Medical Foundation; Mayo School of Health-Related Sciences
Physician Assistant Program
1725 State Street, 4031 Health Science Center
LaCrosse, WI
54601-3767
Phone: (608) 785-8470

http://perth.uwlax.edu/pastudies/

University of Wisconsin, Madison
Physician Assistant Program
Room 1278 Health Sciences Learning Center
750 Highland Avenue
Madison, WI
53705
Phone: (608) 263-5620

http://www.physicianassistant.wisc.edu/

WEST VIRGINIA

Alderson Broaddus College
Physician Assistant Department
PO Box 2036
Philippi, WV
26416
Phone: (304) 457-6283

http://www.ab.edu/academics/degrees/physician_assistant_studies

Mountain State University
Physician Assistant Program
609 South Kanawha Street, PO Box 9003
Beckley, WV
25802-9003
Phone: (304) 253-7351

**http://www.mountainstate.edu/majors/onlinecatalogs/graduate/
programs/PhysiciansAssistant.aspx**